£14.10

Health and the Hunter-Gatherer

Monographs in Human Genetics

Vol. 8

Editors
L. Beckman, Umeå, and M. Hauge, Odense

S. Karger · Basel · München · Paris · London · New York · Sydney

Health and the Hunter-Gatherer

Biomedical Studies on the Hunting and Gathering Populations of Southern Africa

G.T. NURSE and T. JENKINS

Department of Human Genetics, School of Pathology, The South African Institute for Medical Research and University of the Witwatersrand, Johannesburg

8 figures and 26 tables, 1977

S. Karger · Basel · München · Paris · London · New York · Sydney

Monographs in Human Genetics

Vol. 1. Beckman, L. (Uppsala): Isozyme Variations in Man. VIII + 76 p., 33 fig., 22 tab., 1966, ISBN 3-8055-0444-6

Vol. 2. Kjessler, B. (Uppsala): Karyotype, Meiosis and Spermatogenesis in a Sample of Men Attending an Infertility Clinic. VIII + 92 p., 19 fig., 15 tab., 1966. ISBN 3-8055-0445-4

Vol. 3. Morton, Newton, E.; Chung, Chin, S., and Mi, Ming-Pi (Honolulu, Hawaii): Genetics of Interracial Crosses in Hawaii. VIII + 160 p., 5 fig., 42 tab., 1967. ISBN 3-8055-0446-2

Vol. 4. Kirk, R.L. (Canberra): The Haptoglobin Groups in Man. VI + 78 p., 11 fig., 13 tab., 1968. ISBN 3-8055-0447-0

Vol. 5. Giannelli, F. (London): Human Chromosomes DNA Synthesis. VIII + 156 p., 31 fig., 28 tab., 1970. ISBN 3-8055-0448-9

Vol. 6. François, J. (Gent): Aminoacidopathies, Immunoglobinopathies, Neuro-Genetics and Neuro-Ophthalmology. X + 214 p., 26 fig., 49 tab., 1972. ISBN 3-8055-1280-5

Vol. 7. Svejgaard, A.; Hauge, M.; Jersild, C.; Platz, P.; Ryder, L.P.; Staub Nielsen, L. and Thomsen, M. (Copenhagen, Odense): The HLA System. VIII + 104 p., 10 fig., 17 tab., 1975. ISBN 3-8055-2304-1

Cataloging in Publication
Nurse, G.T.
Health and the hunter-gatherer: biomedical studies on the hunting and gathering populations of Southern Africa/G.T. Nurse and T. Jenkins.
(Monographs in human genetics; v. 8)
1. Anthropology, Cultural – Africa, Southern 2. Anthropology, Physical – Africa, Southern 3. Genetics, Population
W1 MO567P v.8/QH 455 N974h
ISBN 3-8055-2401-3

Printed in Switzerland by Buchdruckerei Werner + Bischoff AG, Basel
ISBN 3-8055-2401-3

Contents

Chapter 4. Polymorphisms of No Known Medical Relevance

Chapter 5. Adaptation to the Environment

Chapter 6. Population Structure among the Southern African Hunter-Gatherers

Chapter 7. Conclusions

Preface

This monograph has grown out of the work done over a number of years by a number of workers. It represents a considerable amplification of a paper entitled *Biomedical Studies on Southern African Desert-Dwelling Hunter-Gatherers*, which at the time of writing is due to appear in *Progress in Medical Genetics,* vol. I n.s. (edited by A.G. STEINBERG, A.G. BEARN, B. CHILDS and A. MOTULSKY, and published by W.K. Saunders of Philadelphia). It is not a complete, final and definitive study of the health of the hunting and gathering populations of Southern Africa, but rather an interim report at a critical period in their history. Change is proceeding faster today in Southern Africa than at any time since the *Mfecane* of the early years of the last century when the rise of the Zulu power rippled out in a series of dislodgements of peoples over most of the sub-continent; the process can really only be understood in an historical context broader than we have the scope to give here. What we have tried to do is to describe the biological status of these populations during a particular period, and to present it in a form susceptible to analysis by any interested persons; we have given our own opinions, based on present data, but we make no extravagant claims for their immutability. Most of these data either have appeared, or will appear, in publications whose subjects are more particular than general, though one or two of the more recently investigated populations are described biologically for the first time here.

Southern African history includes the history of three of the major races of mankind. When the first Negroes arrived in the area it was already inhabited by Khoisan ('Capoids', 'Bushmen and Hottentots'); when the first Caucasoids arrived they made contact with Khoisan before they encountered the Negroes. Since then, many of the Khoisan have been absorbed into the Negro and Coloured (mixed) populations, and the unmixed survivors are found mainly in areas where they continue, or continued until recently, to hunt and gather. Their biological individuality is associated with a highly unusual linguistic trait which calls for some explanation, since otherwise the printed forms of their names may appear very strange to the unprepared reader. Khoisan phonology includes a set of consonants known as the 'click sounds', which occur in other languages almost exclusively either as borrowings or as non-verbal exclamations. They are all brief implosive sounds formed at different positions of the tongue: /, the dental click, ǂ, the alveolar, !, the palatal and //, the lateral are all found in the names of populations described here. Fortunately for the printer, the bilabial or 'kiss' click, in which the tongue plays no part, does not, so there is no need to give its symbol. Click sounds may be modified by nasalization or voicing, and each modification constitutes a separate phoneme. There are further peculiarities of Khoisan phonology, but it is not necessary to detail them in the present context. Similar sounds occur in two East African languages, Hadza and Sandawe, which may or may not be Khoisan. As we demonstrate in this monograph, not all the speakers of Khoisan languages are necessarily members of the Khoisan race.

Throughout the work which has gone into the preparation of the monograph, we have been sustained by the groundwork carried out by earlier investigators, and by the support of The South African Institute for Medical Research and the Medical Research Council of South Africa, as well as by the interest and cooperation of the peoples who we were investigating and of our staff. Besides our illustrious Dedicatee, we must acknowledge the friendly help of the late Prof. ISRAEL BERSOHN, Prof. JACK METZ, Prof. J.F. MURRAY, Prof. J.H.S. GEAR, Dr. A. ZOUTENDYK, Prof. HENRY HARPENDING, Prof. PAT DRAPER, Dr. M.C. BOTHA, Mr. W.J. CHASKO jr., Miss ELIZABETH CASHDAN, Dr. ALFRED MERRIWEATHER, Mr. TONY TRAILL, Prof. A.G. STEINBERG, Prof. HERMANN LEHMANN, the staffs of the hospitals and missions of the Kavango Valley, especially those at Andara and Nyangana, the late Dr. JOHANN GILDENHUYS, Dr. STEPHEN GROVÉ, Mr. and Mrs. T. COETZEE and the Rev. and Mrs. F. WEICH of Tsumkwe, Dr. and Mrs. JIRO TANAKA, and the priests and sisters at Aminuis Mission. Without the consistent interest and assistance of Miss CYNTHIA MCINTYRE, Mr. J.L. COHEN and Mr. F. LUBBE of J.L. Cohen Motors, Windhoek, much of our work in South West Africa would have remained undone. The Administration and Hospital Services of South West Africa, and their staff at Tsumkwe, Oshakati, Okombahe, Rundu and Aminuis must also be thanked. We are most grateful to the Botswana Government, and in particular Miss E. WILY, Bushmen Development Officer, for the facilities it has offered us for working in remote parts of that country. Especial thanks are due to the Typing Pool and Mrs. C. MARSCHALL, to the Map Unit and Miss J.R. HARDING, and the Photographic Unit and Mr. and Mrs. M. ULRICH and Mrs. Y. DESCY.

Epistle Dedicatory to Prof. P.V. Tobias

Dear Phillip,

It would not be too much to claim that these pages are as much the outcome of nearly three decades of your work as they are of any process of compilation by us. Without the guiding hand of Tobias, the biological study of the hunter-gatherers of Southern Africa would have been a much more diffuse and formless thing; but you have laboured to bring order and strict observation into a field previously much bedevilled by mythology, and in the process have been able to contribute not only to a geographically limited subject but to the entire study of man. We hope that you will consent to do us the honour of allowing us to dedicate to you this intimation that although much has already been done in this area there remains, as you often remind us, still very much that needs to be done.

We remain,

Your friends and admirers,

George T. Nurse and Trefor Jenkins

Introduction

The hunter-gatherer peoples of the world amount, according to LEE and DEVORE [1968], to 0.001% of the world's population. In absolute numbers, this estimate is of much the same order of magnitude as that they made for the 16th century, when, it is presumed, about 1% of all human beings lived by hunting and gathering. The geographical distribution of such peoples has, however, changed drastically since then. Whereas in the 16th century the entire population of Australia, most of that of North, South and Central America and North-east Asia, and a large proportion of the people of Central and Southern Africa and South-east Asia lived by hunting and gathering, this way of life is now confined to a number of northern circumpolar populations, part of the remaining indigenous peoples of Australia, much the same peoples of South-east Asia as four centuries ago, possibly some South Americans, certainly a number of East Africans, and the inhabitants of the deserts and semi-deserts of Southern Africa.

The popular idea of hunter-gatherers as people engaged in an arduous and unremitting struggle to wrest a precarious living from harsh and forbidding environments depends on several misconceptions. In the first instance, these people may have been led or driven into taking up their present areas of residence by the development of cultures of settlement in those regions which can support such cultures; but we cannot entirely dismiss the possibility that their present situation is the result not of compulsion but of choice. Agriculture and the rearing of livestock make a fuller use of land than dependence on the spontaneous products of that land ever can. There are, however, natural limitations to the extent of the land that is able to support crops or cattle, and on its margin there remain resources which can be utilized by those willing to exploit them. Nor are such resources necessarily sparse. Given a sufficiently low population density, an appropriate hunting technique and/or enough knowledge about food plants and insects, they can provide a subsistence which is more than adequate. It has been shown by MEGGIT [1964], SERVICE [1966], LEE [1965, 1968], TANAKA [1975], and others that food resources are almost always available in quantities ranging from sufficient to abundant.

Much of this well-being naturally depends on the narrowness of the range of demand. Before the Neolithic Revolution, when the whole of humanity consisted of hunter-gatherers [COLE, 1970], all of the spontaneous product of the most fertile parts of the world was available. Communities could settle in one place and subsist very well on what could be garnered from the immediate neighbourhood. HARLAN [1967] has demonstrated that the wild wheat of Asia Minor could still support localized settlements of moderate size. What impetus led to the commencement of agriculture is not clear; it may have been a consequence of population growth beyond tolerable levels in such settlements. Such a development could have led also to eventually successful attempts to breed as livestock animals which had hitherto been hunted as prey. The choice must have arisen between staying in the same place but changing the way of life, and keeping the life-style but moving elsewhere; this choice would have faced a succession of hunter-gatherers ever since, until now, with the greater part of the cultivable world settled, they are confined to what appear to us as inhospitable environments. There must have been countless opportunities for the forebears of the modern hunter-gatherers to adopt a culture of settlement; such opportunities still exist, even in as crowded a world as the present; but there have always been some who have rejected them and pressed outwards beyond the margins.

It is in some ways easy to comprehend the motives for such decisions. Cultivation and cattle-rearing demand systematic effort and planning, and place their practitioners at the mercy of the elements. They involve voluntary limitations of resources and often a good deal of hard physical work, generally at particular times of the year. Hunting and gathering make use of a wide range of resources in the availability of some of which there may be seasonal variation but all of which are usually routinely available at one time or another. The hunter-gatherer finds his food more fortuitously; there is not need for complex planning, and when supplies fail there is nothing to keep him in any particular place. The culture of settlement, in short, imposes a pattern of demands more extensive than that found in hunting and gathering. Discontent arises when demands are frustrated; the fewer there are the more likely they are to be satisfied. The settled life is in many ways the harder and more precarious, and that of the hunter-gatherer the more stable and less arduous. In fact, SAHLINS [1968] has described it as affluent.

Of course there have been, and still are, intermediate stages between hunting and gathering and the culture of husbandry. It is sometimes difficult to decide where hunting and gathering ceases and the settled life begins. Nomads with herds, whose men hunt and whose women gather wild vegetables, or even villagers with gardens but without cattle and dependent on hunting and to some extent on gathering, would appear to qualify in part. The Gypsies of Western Europe seem to satisfy many of the criteria for hunter-gatherers but not to be regarded as such. Perhaps a lack of dependence on trade is a prerequisite for the genuine hunting and gathering life. The fact remains that no satisfactory definition of this way of life resulted from the conference of Man the Hunter held in Chicago in 1965 [LEE and DEVORE, 1968] or has been proposed since.

The hunter-gatherers of Southern Africa exist in a variety of groups not all of whom are biologically interrelated. They are, in fact, divided between two major biological races, Khoisan and Negro; though there has been a considerable flow of Khoisan genes into the settled Bantu-speaking Negro populations [JENKINS, 1972], there is evidence of only a small degree of gene exchange between Negro and Khoisan hunter-gatherers, even in those populations which have recently adopted a culture of settlement. This is all the more surprising inasmuch as many of the hunter-gatherer groups, including the Negroes, speak Khoisan languages. The main exceptions to this are the Kwisi and the Cimba, whose languages are Bantu and shared with Negro neighbours. The Kgalagadi language is certainly Bantu, but sufficiently remote from Tswana not to be classifiable as a dialect of that language. It is obvious that there must be some reason for so curious and unexpected a phenomenon, and investigations aimed at elucidating it continue.

This major human biological interface is of particular interest insofar as members of both races in places share a common ecosystem and a common material culture. In consequence, it may become possible, once the mass of accumulated serogenetic and biomedical data has been properly analyzed, to draw rather more conclusions about the influence of the environment on certain of the polymorphisms than we are able to do as yet.

The Southern African hunter-gatherer groups are in the main desert-dwelling. One can claim this with all the more assurance since there is no satisfactory definition of a desert. As a geographical term, the word is usually applied to any barren and sparsely inhabitated area of large size. The Encyclopaedia Britannica (1951) describes a desert as a land 'which produces insufficient vegetation to support a human population'. It seems to be requisite that surface water should be absent or only seasonally present [BURTON, 1974], and that such precipitation as occurs should not contribute to a sea or an ocean. Deserts often are inhabited, and it might be more accurate to expand the Encyclopaedia Britannica definition to refer only to settled populations.

Chapter 1. The Southern African Deserts and their Inhabitants

The Deserts of Southern Africa

Three deserts are universally recognized in Southern Africa. A fourth, the Great Karroo in the interior of the Cape Province of the Republic of South Africa, though it would meet most of the requirements for being a desert, supports quite a large settled population. It is in any case no longer inhabited by any hunter-gatherers, and would consequently be excluded from the terms of this account. The three which remain are the Kalahari Desert, extending east to west from the south-western border of Rhodesia to the fertile uplands of central South West Africa and from the neighbourhood of the Zambesi and Kavango rivers in the north to the margin of the Karroo in the south; the Namib Desert, a strip averaging 80 miles wide along the coast of South West Africa; and the Moçâmedes Desert in south-western Angola. The last-named is virtually a northward prolongation of the Namib (fig. 1, table I).

The Namib is a sandy desert. To the south of the Kuiseb River, there is an area of enormous shifting dunes, though in its southernmost part, between the Lüderitz railway and the Orange River, the surface is hard and in places broken by rocky plugs. Smaller dunes extend northwards from the Kuiseb to the Swakop River, and north of the Swakop the surface is again hard and crossed by rock dykes. Part of it is involved in an extension of the Kaokoveld lava bed [WELLINGTON, 1967], and at this northern end and for some way to the south of it no very definite demarcation exists between the Namib and the almost equally desert-like Kaokoveld and the Brandberg massif. For the rest of its extent the desert is bounded on the east by a great escarpment, on the plateaux to the east of which lie the agricultural and grazing areas of South West Africa.

The Moçâmedes Desert to the north of the Kunene River shows much the same features as the Namib and shares a similarly sparse vegetation of low karroo succulents, cucurbits and patches of hardy grasses. The extraordinary *Welwitschia bainesii,* a gymnosperm tree with a subterraneous trunk, is common, and unique, to both deserts. There are more dunes along the Moçâmedes coast than there are in the northern Namib, and the interior is flatter and extends further inland. The port of Moçâmedes marks almost the northernmost limit of the desert.

The great Kalahari Desert lies in a central basin in the southern-most of the coalescing plateaux which make up most of the interior of Southern and East Africa. It occupies the greater part of Botswana, and extends into the northern Cape Province. Most of the eastern quarter of South West Africa is Kalahari, and in the arid southern part of that country its boundaries are difficult to fix. It consists broadly of a surface layer of unconsolidated sand overlying consolidated calcareous sand and gravel and relieved at rare intervals by sandstone outcrops [WELLINGTON, 1967]. In the southern part the surface is flat, though long dunes are found towards the middle and generally lie parallel to the dry watercourses. There is good vegetation cover

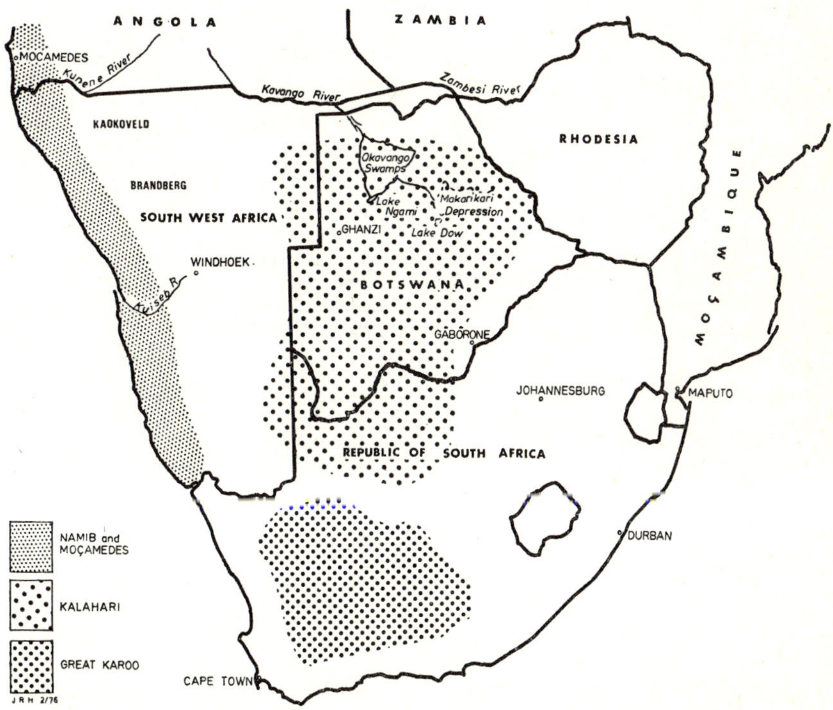

Fig. 1. The deserts of Southern Africa; their margins are fluctuant, due to variations in rainfall. Shown here is their approximate minimum extent.

Table I. Key to maps and tables

Population	Alternative name	No. on map	Reference	Ref. in ta
San	Bushmen			
!Kung, of Angola (E)	Sekele, Cassequeles	4	Almeida [1954]	3
!Kung, of Angola (W)	Kwankhwala, Mucuancalas	5	Almeida [1954]	3
!Kung, of Kavango	Northern Bushmen	3	Zoutendyk *et al.* [1953]	2
	G!äg!ai	27	Jenkins *et al.* [in preparation]	10
!Kung, unspecified	Kung	1	Pijper [1932]	1
		20	Jenkins *et al.* [1963]	8
!Kung, northern		21	Jenkins [1972]	6
!Kung, Ngami		22	Jenkins [1972]	6
!Kung, Dobe		23	Jenkins [1972]	6
!Kung, /ai/ai		24	Jenkins [1972]	6
!Kung, /du/da		25	Jenkins [1972]	6
!Kung, Tsumkwe		26	Jenkins, [1972]	6
			Jenkins *et al.* [1974]	17
//au//en	Auen	2	Pijper [1932]	1
		19	Jenkins [1972]	6
Nharo	Central San	6	Tobias and Zoutendyk, quoted by Tobias [1966]	4
		6	Weiner and Zoutendyk [1959]	5
	Naron	18	Jenkins [1972]	6
G/wi		16	Jenkins *et al.* [1975]	7
G//ana		17	Jenkins *et al.* [1975]	7
!Xõ	Southern San	13	Jenkins [1972]	6
	Magong	7	Weiner and Zoutendyk [1959]	5
		14	Jenkins and Nurse [1976]	16
ǂhuã:		15	Nurse, Traill and Jenkins [in preparation]	13
G!aokx'ate		36	Jenkins, Botha and Nurse [in preparation]	10
Khoi	Hottentots			
Kede	Muquedes	9	Almeida [1954]	3
Hei//om	Heikum	8	Pijper [1932]	1
		30	Jenkins, Botha and Nurse [in preparation]	10
Topnaar, Sesfontein		29	Jenkins [1972]	6
Topnaar, Kuiseb		28	Jenkins and Brain [1967]	9
Nama of Keetmanshoop		37	Nurse and Jenkins [1974]	18
Negro				
Kwengo of Angola	Zama, Cazamas	10	Almeida [1954]	3
Kwengo of Caprivizipfel	Barakwengo, Kxoe	33	Nurse and Jenkins [in preparation]	14
Kwisi	Mucuisses	11	Almeida [1954]	3
Kwadi	Mucuepes, Curocas	12	Almeida [1954]	3
Cimba	Tjimba, Ovatjimba	32	Jenkins, Gildenhuys and Nurse [in preparation]	–
Dama	Damara, Bergdama	31	Knussmann [1969]	11
			[illegible] [1969/70]	11
		31	Nurse *et al.* [1975]	12
Kgalagadi		34	Jenkins *et al.* [1968]	8
Denasena		35	Chasko *et al.* [in preparation]	15

here, and in places it is even possible to speak of 'forests' of low dry thorn trees. The nature of the Kalahari formation, with the centre lying at a lower altitude than the northern margin, leads to the presence in the northern part of some considerable areas of open water, such as Lakes Ngami and Dow and the swamps into which the large Kavango River drains. In a good wet season, surface water is plentiful; the numerous shallow pans with beds of hardened crystalline salts fill with water, and the swamp drainage area overflows into the large Makarikari Depression (fig. 1). For most of the year, however, only underground water is available, and the human and other inhabitants depend on the moisture they can dig to or get from the vegetation.

The Kalahari experiences an abrupt annual rainy season of short duration, but precipitation in the Namib and the Moçâmedes consists almost entirely of condensation from sea mists produced by the cold off-shore Benguela current. This naturally affects both the variety and the quantity of the flora and fauna. Large game is present in the Kalahari, in places quite abundantly, while in the other two deserts it is confined to a few species of antelope, which are hardly ever seen. In all three deserts, there are several thriving species of rodents, though the species found in the Kalahari differ from those along the coast. There are also pronounced differences in the bird and insect life.

Desert-Dwelling Human Populations

The rarity of surface water in these deserts precludes agriculture, except where irrigation from boreholes is practised. Animal husbandry is barely possible; goats, donkeys and horses, all recent introductions, are found in some places in the Kalahari, and bovine cattle can be reared with care in a few selected locations. There are patches of settlement around pumps and boreholes installed either by private individuals or by governments, and these 'oases' are often occupied and controlled by European settlers. This is particularly the case in the middle sector of the eastern part of South West Africa, and in Ghanzi District in Botswana (fig. 1) [cf. SILBERBAUER, 1965]. The occasional farm, drawing its water from a borehole, can even be found in the Namib. For the rest, the resources of the deserts are made use of only by hunter-gatherer populations. Some of these are now being induced to settle, usually with government encouragement and assistance, as at Okambahe and Tsumkwe in South West Africa and Bere in Botswana; some spend part of the year at settlements and the rest in their traditional way of life, and this applies to part of the Tsumkwe population; others have taken to a dependent life, either as clients of settled Negroes [SILBERBAUER and KUPER, 1966] or as labourers on the farms around Ghanzi in Botswana or near Grootfontein, Gobabis and Tsumeb in South West Africa (fig. 1).

The San

The best known and most numerous of the hunter-gatherer peoples of Southern Africa are the San or 'Bushmen'. By convention they are divided as three linguistic groups, a Northern, a Central and a Southern [BLEEK, 1927]. The cultural differences among these groups are minimal. Though some genetic markers tend to show a cline with latitude, this is not useful for distinguishing the speakers of Central Bushmen. Of all the peoples still extant in Southern Africa, the San seem to have the best claim to antiquity of residence. It appears that they once extended over a considerable part of the rest of the continent; there are skeletal remains from East Africa which closely resemble the 'proto-Bushman' skeletons found in South Africa [WELLS, 1952a, b], and there is good evidence that at some time during the Later Stone Age – which of course for them persisted into the present century [STOW, 1905] – they were distributed over a good deal of Southern and East Africa [TOBIAS, 1960].

Until quite recently, it appeared that they were dwindling towards extinction; COON [1955] was under the impression that they comprised only a few hundred individuals, but in the same year TOBIAS [1955a], with rather more reliable data at his disposal, estimated their numbers at about 53,000. Probably more than half live in Botswana. They are widely scattered over that country, except in the extreme south-east and to the east of the series of villages along the railway line, and include representatives of all three main language groups and possibly of a fourth [TRAILL, 1973]. They are usually thinly spread, as one would expect of a desert population, and could amount to rather more than the 24,652 enumerated in the 1964 census. SILBERBAUER [1965] estimates that figure as probably too low by about 20%, owing to the difficulties of ascertainment and the number culturally accepted as Negroes. In South West Africa, the San are somewhat more accessible, but it seems unlikely that the 1970 Census, which gives a total of 21,909, includes them all. Surprisingly little is known of the smaller groups, particularly those reputed to inhabit or to have inhabited the central and southern section of the Namib desert. Their names have been recorded [SCHA-

PERA, 1930] and accounts of their approximate geographical locations collated [NURSE, 1972], but if they do still exist they are extraordinarily elusive. The only San populations known for certain to be present in the south of the country are those who live in the Aminuis Reserve, where they still hunt and gather, or are settled on the desert farms adjoining it. These include almost all the surviving G!aokx'ate and a number of Nharo. In the centre of the northern part of the country, where the Kalahari shades off into the Kaokoveld, and in the Etosha Game Reserve, there are still hunter-gatherer bands. The Strandlopers of the northern Namib, long thought to be extinct, have been re-identified in a party which has come up from the coast and settled at Sesfontein in the Kaokoveld. The largest concentration of San, if concentration it can be called, is in the north-east of the country. It consists mainly of various subdivisions of the Zhu/oasi or !Kung, and is continuous with similar populations in north-western Botswana and southern Angola.

All, or almost all, the San in Angola belong to this large group. Their

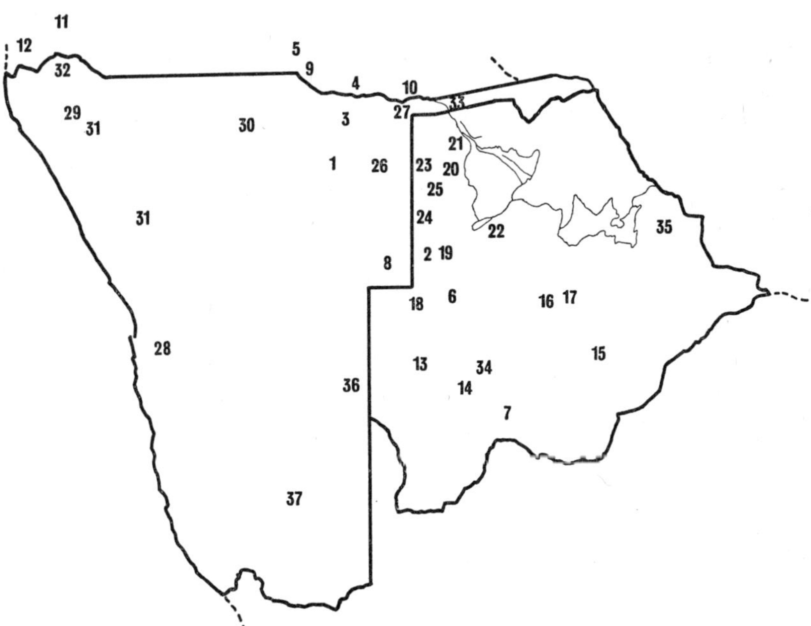

Fig. 2. The locations of the hunter-gatherer populations discussed. Since some of the populations are migrant, the locations are necessarily only approximate. The key to the identities of the populations is provided in table I.

numbers were estimated by Estermann [1956] as probably in excess of 5,000, but Guerreiro [1968] considers that 6,000 would be a very conservative figure and believes that 10,000 might be nearer the mark. It must not be forgotten, though, that Portuguese writers classify the Kwengo as San [Almeida, 1965]. With the exception of those who live in the south-west of the country, they inhabit forest areas with abundant water, and can hardly be said to be desert-dwellers. Both divisions of the true San in Angola, the Kwankhala and the Sekele as they are called by their Bantu-speaking neighbours, do, however, have contacts with the !Kung-speakers to the south, and their way of life appears to be very similar [Ribas, n.d.].

There are San bands in the Kalahari Gemsbok Park on the borders of South Africa, Botswana and South West Africa, and there are certainly a number of San still resident in the South African parts of the Kalahari, though they prefer to be regarded as Tswana and little is known of their present numbers [Breutz, 1963]. We have personally encountered San individuals in paid employment in the northern Cape Province; these live scattered and unobtrusive lives among the preponderant Negroes and Coloureds, who are, in fact or purportedly, of mixed race. In the eastern Transvaal a single very small band on the verge of extinction can still be found near Lake Chrissie [Potgieter, 1955]. There are no figures, reliable or otherwise, available to us about the numbers of San in Rhodesia or Zambia. It seems doubtful whether they are true San; they adjoin the Khoisan-speaking Negro hunter-gatherers of northern Botswana, and may well represent branches of the same peoples.

The Khoi

Hunting and gathering are not usually part of the Khoi ('Hottentot') way of life, though some groups, and most notably the Saan of the Namib, have practised them. By far the largest number of Khoi live in South West Africa, under the name of Nama, including not only the original Nama of the country but also peoples who migrated thither from the Cape during the 18th and early 19th centuries. The archetypal Khoi hunter-gatherers are no longer to be found, though the semi-settled groups in the Kuiseb Valley and the Kaokoveld hunt and gather in the adjacent desert. Out of the total of about 33,000 Nama in South West Africa, these probably constitute about 3% at the most. The present authors incline to agree with Redinha [1974] and Botha [personal commun.], and will give additional reasons for this below, in regarding the Hei//om hunter-gatherers, who are usually called 'Bushmen', as Khoi. The Hei//om live in northern South West Africa, mainly around the Etosha Pan and eastwards along the fringes of the true Kalahari. Some have scattered into the forests to the north and there are reports of a few bands in Angola. The only available estimate of their numbers talks of 'a few or several thousand' [BOTHA *et al.*, 1973]. REDINHA mentions 'Hottentots' in southern Angola in addition to Hei//om, near Ruacaná on the Kunene River, but refers to them as a '*grupo diminuto*'. ESTERMANN [1956] doubts whether there are any more Khoi in Angola than can be accounted for by the servants brought by migrant White South African nomad pastoralists and left behind by them. Both ESTERMANN and REDINHA count the small surviving group of Kede hunter-gatherers as Khoi, and WESTPHAL [1971] regards their language as related to Hei//om.

The Nama extend into the western parts of Botswana, but not in any great numbers, and there are still some occasionally met with in the northern Cape Province. A more considerable, but still sparse and rapidly disappearing, Khoi population consists of the !Ora or Korana of the Orange River Valley. All of these are settled or in employment, and outside the purview of this account. The Griqua, who are often described as Khoi because they preserve some traces of Khoi language and customs, are more properly included among the hybrid populations which constitute the Cape Coloureds [NURSE and JENKINS, 1975; NURSE, 1975].

Negro Hunter-Gatherers

Whereas the majority of the San are hunter-gatherers, and hunting and gathering are still to a greater or lesser degree practised by an appreciable proportion of the Khoi, the Negroes almost everywhere in Africa have adopted a culture of settlement, often involving mixed farming and occasionally flowering into a high degree of urban civilization. Negro populations probably settled later in Southern Africa than in the rest of sub-Saharan Africa. Their migrations southward may well have occurred first as a movement of people who rejected new-fangled settlement in favour of traditional hunting and gathering. Certainly, the Dama and Kgalagadi, the two Negro groups reputed to be the most anciently settled south of the Kunene and the Zambesi, still include hunter-gatherers.

The Kgalagadi speak a Tswana-related language and are found mostly along the fringes of the Kalahari, into which they are said to have retreated following the arrival of the second Negro immigrant wave represented by the ancestors of the modern Rolong and Tlhaping. Their way of life has until recently greatly resembled that of the San, even to the extent of patron-client relationships with settled Negro populations [SCHAPERA, 1953]. Their numbers are difficult to estimate, though they probably run into several thousands.

The origins of the Dama of South West Africa have posed a riddle to several generations of researchers. They are a numerous people, estimated in the 1970 Census as about 65,000. Morphologically and serologically they are undoubtedly Negro [KNUSSMANN, 1969; NURSE *et al.*, 1976], though the language they speak is Nama. Until the last century, a proportion were held in slavery by the Nama and the Herero and the rest led a hunting-gathering life. The latter still continues in places, particularly around the Brandberg, but permanent and independent settlement, and employment in the towns, now make up the way of life of the majority of the Dama.

A resemblance to the Dama has been claimed for the Negro hunter-gatherer peoples of the Moçâmedes Desert. Of the Kuroka, Kwepe or Kwadi, who speak a click language which WESTPHAL [1971] regards tentatively as possibly related to Nama and Central Bush, only a single small band remains [ESTERMANN, 1956; ALMEIDA, 1965; REDINHA, 1974]. REDINHA classes the Kwadi and Kwisi together under the name Vatua, by which they are known to their Bantu-speaking neighbours, and which ESTERMANN uses as a collective term (embracing the Dama) for Negro hunter-gatherers. The Kwisi speak a Bantu language, Kuvale, but no study has yet determined whether they have their own dialect of it. They are more numerous than the Kwadi, and REDINHA states that in 1960 they were estimated at more than 5,000. Not all live in the desert.

In addition to the Dama, two other Khoisan-speaking Negro groups have been studied. The so-called 'Black Bushmen', the Central Bush-speaking Kwengo or Barakwengo of north-western Botswana and the western Caprivizipfel, the corridor extending eastwards from the far north-eastern corner of South West Africa, have been shown to resemble their immediate neighbours the undoubtedly Negro Mbukushu too closely for them to continue to be regarded as San [NURSE and JENKINS, in preparation]. The Kwengo are a group continuous with the Zama or Cazama of south-eastern Angola, who share their morphological characters and appearance. As this study shows, the physical resemblance to the Mbukushu is borne out by close serological similarities to Negroes, and the Kwengo must be accounted Negro. Much the same applies to much of the 'Sarwa' population of northern Botswana. The name 'Mosarwa' is the Tswana for a Bushman; it is not confined to the

San, and appears to relate to a way of life rather than to have any biological meaning. The Sarwa from north-eastern Botswana who have been studied give strong indications of being biologically Negro rather than San. For convenience of reference here they will be referred to as Denasena, a name occasionally applied to them.

A small number of Cimba, a Herero-speaking Negro people which hunts and gathers, are to be found in the Kaokoveld and across the border in Angola. According to VAN WARMELO [1962] they represent a population which has had to abandon the pastoralism of their Himba neighbours, with whom they are otherwise identical, on account of their having lost their cattle by sickness or theft. In common with the Kwisi, for whom this is also claimed [ESTERMANN, 1956], they could consequently be one of the rather rare examples of a reversion to hunting and gathering after a period of settlement [cf. LÉVI-STRAUSS, 1952]. There are probably less than 100 Cimba in all. MACCALMAN and GROBBELAAR [1965] consider them quite distinct from the Himba; so does VAN DER MERWE [1969a, b].

The Negro population of South and South West Africa, Botswana and Angola amounts altogether to about 23 million. The total numbers of Negro hunter-gatherers cannot be more than 25,000, most of them Dama, Kwisi and Denasena and related groups.

Chapter 2. The Physical Characters of the Southern African Hunter-Gatherers

A good proportion of the anthropological work done on the hunting and gathering peoples of Southern Africa has consisted of studies of their gross morphology. The large studies of the Khoi by VON LUSCHAN [1907], of the Nharo and //au//en San ('Naron' and 'Auen') by TOBIAS [1955b; 1956a, b], of the /?auni-ǂKhomani San by DART [1937], of the Nama Khoi by SCHULTZE [1928] and WELLS [1952a, b] and of the Negro Dama by KNUSSMANN and KNUSSMANN [1969/70], as well as those of the !Kung San of LEBZELTER [1931] and WELLS [1952a, b], are probably the most noteworthy. Smaller series of importance are those of FISCHER [1913] on a handful of Nama, of GROBBELAAR [1956] on the Korana Khoi, of TOERIEN [1958] on the //xegwi San of Lake Chrissie, of GALLOWAY [1937] and TOBIAS [1955b] on small Khoi groups, and the three (!) Strandlopers described but not measured by DART [1955]. There are earlier, rather impressionistic and anecdotal accounts of the physique of both San and Khoi in FRITSCH [1872], DORNAN [1922], SCHULTZE [1907] and PASSARGE [1908], and in numerous travel narratives, of which GALTON's [1853] is that which comes closest to constituting a scientific appraisal. These have recently been reviewed and summarized by HITZEROTH [1972]. There have been several dermatoglyphic studies on the San [CUMMINS, 1955; TOBIAS, 1961] and Khoi [FLEISCHHACKER, 1934], and claims have been made for the anthropological value of this system [RIFE, 1953]. Though it appears to distinguish among the linguistic groups of the San, its genetic basis is not clear enough for any distinct conclusions to be drawn, and it is doubtful whether it has any physiological function. The gross physical characters have lately tended to be underesteemed in genetic studies, largely because of their complex and usually polygenic mode of inheritance and the consequent difficulty of assessing their value as genetic markers; but a large part of human physiology is conditioned by the morphological conformation of man, and no biomedical survey can properly ignore it.

The Morphology of the San

According to TOBIAS [1960, 1972], the San may be characterized as small of stature, possessed of postural peculiarities, most notably a lumbar lordosis, and having isolated fat deposits over the thighs (steatomeria) and buttocks (steatopygia) [KRUT and SINGER, 1963]. Their skin colour is a light yellowish-brown; skin reflectance studies by WEINER *et al.* [1964] showed the San to be the lightest in colour of the unmixed indigenous peoples of Southern Africa. Their head hair tends to consist of tightly spiralled tufts ('peppercorns'), and their eyes are often slanting, with prominent epicanthic or other folds. They have unusually small and commonly lobeless ears, the helices of which are very frequently overrolled. Their noses are broad and their faces small, flattish and orthognathic, contrasting markedly with the prognathic faces of Negroes. The tablier, macronymphia or 'Hottentot apron', a lengthening and hypertrophy of the labia minora, is prominent in some women [DE VILLIERS, 1961], while many men manifest ithyphally, or horizontal projection of the non-erect penis [DRURY and DRENNAN, 1926]. A number of infantile or 'paedomorphic' features are evident in the head and skull of the San. They have a 'lower frequency of prodontism (dental prognathism), of Carabelli tubercles on the upper first molars and shovel-shaped incisors, less frequent overbite and more common underbite, a higher incidence of spaced teeth and a rather lower incidence of well-accommodated teeth in both the upper and lower jaws' [TOBIAS, 1972] than the South African Negroes. Their skulls tend to be pentagonal and relatively broad, with bossing in the frontal region, small but definite glabella and absent or only weakly present supraciliary ridges. The cheek-bones are prominent and the chin fairly pointed and rounded.

The body is slender, the limbs are thin and not heavily muscled. The upper extremity is short in comparison with the lower, and the hands and feet are small; both extremities are short compared to the body. In pubescent girls, the areola of the nipple becomes very swollen, so as almost to resemble a ball resting at the apex of the breast; though this wanes with the suckling of the first child, the areola does remain unusually prominent until sagging of the breasts sets in. The deep and early wrinkling of the skin of the San is particularly noticeable on the face and abdomen. There is little subcutaneous fat generally, though San receiving a high-calorie diet over a long period can become noticeably chubby.

The Morphology of the Khoi

Few morphological differences have been noted between the Khoi and the San except in overall size. There seems to be a tendency for the head and face of the Khoi to be slightly longer and for the bridge of the nose to be more prominent. SCHULTZE [1928] believed the physical characteristics possessed in common by San and Khoi to be too numerous for them to be regarded as separate races, and this claim has never yet been refuted by classical physical anthropological or any other methods. DRENNAN [1929] found the dental differences to be minimal. In 1911, PERINGUEY concluded that it was 'well-nigh impossible to distinguish now from outer appearance a so-called Colonial Bushman from a native of Hottentot origin', and went on to suggest that right since the beginning of European settlement at the Cape the distinction had been arbitrarily made. 'Those who had herds of cattle, and were not too small, were Hottentots; the others, who lived mostly by the chase or kept no cattle or sheep, and were small, were Boschiesmen.' The position is complicated by the undoubted fact that the Khoi have at some time received an appreciable contribution of Caucasoid genes; some of this has certainly resulted from Dutch and British settlement, though it has been suggested that admixture originally occurred in north-east Africa before the Khoi migrated southwards [FISCHER, 1913; SCHAPERA, 1926]. FRITSCH [1872], who had an earlier opportunity than many physical anthropologists to examine the Khoi, comments on the number of their similarities to the Bushmen and, like many 19th-century writers, discusses the tablier at great length. There is no published account of the presence or absence of ithyphally among the Khoi.

The Morphology of the Negroes

There have been no classical physical anthropological studies on any desert-dwelling Negro population with the exception of those of the KNUSSMANNS [1969, 1969/70] on the Dama. A few morphological particulars, mostly impressions, may be gathered from the Portuguese writers. ESTERMANN [1956] states that there is no pronounced somatic difference between the Kwisi and their Kuvale neighbours, but that the Kwadi or Kuroka do not appear typically Negro but possess some unspecified Khoisan traits. According to ALMEIDA [1965], the latter are of tall stature, spiral-haired, with flat broad noses and thick lips, and not easily distinguishable from the

Kuvale, Kwanyoka and Himba, the Negro groups with which they come in closest contact. The KNUSSMANNS [1969/70] have published a set of seven somatic measurements of the Dama, and these show them to fall into the general Negro range.

The Negroes are on average of medium height, with the sitting height approximately half, and the span greater than, the stature. They are dark of skin; when they have not received any admixture of genes, they can be very dark. They have hair which is black, woolly and of fine to medium texture, and do not commonly show eye obliquity or eye folds. The Negro ear is of moderate size with no marked helix overrolling and with a usually free and well-developed lobe. The moderately broad nasal bridge is slightly raised and straight in profile, in contrast to the concavity often found in the Khoisan. Prognathism is pronounced, and there is a high prevalence of median diastema. In general, Negroes have ovoid, proportionately long skulls, with well-marked glabellae and superciliary ridges and little or no frontal bossing. Their cheek-bones are moderately prominent, and only rarely are their chins pointed.

The occasional finding of tablier and steatopygia in the women is most common in those groups which have received a large Khoisan admixture or which practise artificial elongation of the labia minora. The breasts tend to be more rounded and regular in contour than those of Khoisan women, and the areolae, though large, are not distinctive. Negroes are generally of muscular build, with rounded limbs and, except in times of famine or in extreme old age, do not show much wrinkling of the skin. Moderate deposits of subcutaneous fat are usual.

Sero-Genetic Studies on Southern African Hunter-Gatherers to 1966

It is now about ten years since TOBIAS [1966] reviewed the total published data on sero-genetic studies of the peoples of Africa south of the Sahara. The intervening period has seen a considerable increase in the number of systems which can be investigated, and it seems convenient to use that year as a watershed in these studies. Most of the sero-genetic data on Southern African hunter-gatherers up to that time are shown in tables II–V, which consist of material from PIJPER [1932], ZOUTENDYK *et al.* [1953], ALMEIDA [1954], BARNICOT *et al.* [1959], WEINER and ZOUTENDYK [1958, 1959] and the unpublished work of TOBIAS and ZOUTENDYK [1958, 1959] detailed in TOBIAS [1966]. Care has been taken to consider only hunter-gatherer populations,

Table II. Sero-genetic studies on Southern African hunter-gatherers before 1966: the ABO system

Population	n	Phenotypes				Gene frequencies			χ^2[1]
		A	AB	B	O	*A*	*B*	*O*	
San									
Kung[1]	268	75	10	21	162	0.163	0.060	0.777	4.96
Auen[1]	280	87	27	15	151	0.188	0.078	0.734	53.44
Northern[2]	446	151	7	38	250	0.197	0.052	0.751	0.64
'Cassequeles'[3]	605	202	27	26	350	0.194	0.045	0.761	31.84
'Mucuancualas'[3]	814	271	100	56	387	0.209	0.101	0.690	154.20
Central[4]	82	18	2	2	60	0.120	0.025	0.855	5.21
Central[5]	114	40	0	4	70	0.196	0.018	0.788	1.00
'Magon'[5]	72	25	0	3	44	0.198	0.021	0.781	0.75
Khoi									
Heikum[1]	67	20	5	10	32	0.190	0.119	0.691	1.67
'Muquedes'[3]	62	23	8	4	27	0.288	0.102	0.660	11.11
Negro									
'Cazamas'[3]	239	76	11	20	132	0.205	0.076	0.719	5.54
'Mucuisses'[3]	179	78	16	21	64	0.293	0.109	0.598	2.65
'Mucuepes'[3]	45	19	12	2	12	0.314	0.170	0.516	16.43

The 'Cassequeles' and 'Mucuancualas' are the two divisions (Sekele and Kwankhala) into which the adjoining Negroes place the !Kung of Angola [ALMEIDA, 1965]. The 'Cazamas' are the Zama or Kwengo, the 'Mucuisses' are the Kwisi, the 'Muquedes' the Kede and the 'Mucuepes' the Kwadi, or Kuroka. That orthographic idiosyncracy is not confined to Portuguese writers is shown by the 'Auen', or //au//en, and the 'Magong', or !Xõ. In justice to these writers, it must be stated that the simpler forms were chosen out of consideration for the comfort of their readers, a courtesy which the present authors through pedantry withhold.

Table III. Sero-genetic studies on southern African hunter-gatherers before 1966: rhesus and V

Population	n	Phenotypes					Gene frequencies				χ^2 (rhesus)	d.f.
		ccDee	CDee	ccDE	CDE	V+	R^0	R^1	R^2	V		
San												
Northern[2]	232	183	40	9	0	–	0.888	0.092	0.020	–	0.98	1
Central[5]	114	77	32	5	0	6	0.822	0.156	0.022	0.027	0.95	1
Central[4]	31	–	–	–	–	4	–	–	–	0.067	–	–
Southern[4]	72	–	–	–	–	3	–	–	–	0.021	–	–

for which reason the Khoi samples of PIJPER [1935] and ZOUTENDYK *et al.* [1955], which represent settled communities, have not been included. Some studies which comprised undifferentiated samples, and whose value for purposes of comparison was thereby reduced, have been omitted. Dr. A. ZOUTENDYK has kindly allowed us access to his original work-sheets so that resorting could be carried out, but since all the members except 14 of his

Table IV. Sero-genetics studies on Southern African hunter-gatherers before 1966: MNS and Henshaw

Population	n	Phenotypes										Gene frequencies					χ^2	d.f.
		MMS	MMss	MNS	MNSHe	MNss	MNssHe	NNS	NNSHe	NNss	NNssHe	*MS*	*Ms*	*NS*	*Ns*	*NsHe*		
San																		
Northern[2]	188	14	57	12	2	66	0	2	1	33	1	0.068	0.522	0.023	0.369	0.018	16.09	1
Central[4]	79	31			34				14				0.608		0.392			

Table V. Sero-genetic studies on Southern African hunter-gatherers before 1966: various blood group systems

Population	n	Phenotypes						Gene frequencies			
		Duffy Fy(a+)	Kell K+	PP_1^+	Lutheran Lu(a+)	Diego Di(a+)	Sutter Js(a+)	Fy^a	P^1	Js^a	K
San											
Northern[2]	108	17	–	–	–	–	–	0.082	–	–	–
Northern[2]	106	–	11	–	–	–	–	–	–	–	0.053
Northern[2]	89	–	–	–	0	–	–	–	–	–	–
Central[4]	68	19	–	34	–	–	–	0.151	0.293	–	–
Central[4]	31	–	–	–	–	0	–	–	–	–	–
Central[5]	114	–	–	–	–	0	6	–	–	0.027	–
Southern (Magon)[4]	72	–	–	–	–	0	3	–	–	0.021	–

large sample were !Kung from the Kavango area, and the internal agreement for ABO and rhesus was so good, these 14 individuals have been retained. The unsatisfactory internal agreement for MNSs Henshaw can probably be ascribed to the poor quality of the anti-S serum available in the early 1950s. Gene frequencies and, where possible, χ^2 for homogeneity, have been re-calculated for all the observed data. Despite the fact that in the Zoutendyk *et al.* [1953] and Weiner and Zoutendyk [1959] samples weak A groups were detected, and recorded, in the ABO system, this is not reflected in table II, where a pooled A is shown to make the series more comparable with the other, less sophisticated, ones. In this we have followed the precedent of Tobias [1966].

We have not been able to find any data for the Angolan desert-dwellers on any other system than ABO, and the investigations of other systems in Southern African desert-dwellers had, up to that time, been carried out only on San. Two populations had been investigated for variation in the rhesus, MN, and Duffy systems; one of those had been tested also for the presence of the K antigen in the Kell system and Lu(a) in the Lutheran system and Js(a) in the Sutter system. One population had been tested for the two last-named antigens only. These results are shown in table V. Investigation of the heritable variation in haptoglobin and transferrin patterns had likewise been carried out on only one population. In a group of 113 San, examined at Ghanzi and described as 'central', Barnicot *et al.* [1959] found 12 to have the haptoglobin 1 phenotype, 40 to be 2–1, none to be 2–1 mod, 59 to be haptoglobin 2, and 2 to be anhaptoglobinaemic. One member of the same sample was a transferrin D_1 homozygote, 99 were C homozygotes, and 13 were CD_1. Three populations, one described as 'central', one as 'central, south of the Okavango' and the third as 'miscellaneous central' had been investigated without success for variation in haemoglobin types [GRIFFITHS, 1953].

By 1966, the major period of morphological examination of these peoples was substantially over, and the age of serological investigation had commenced. The foregoing account will have shown that the principal direction of the enquiries up till then had been anthropological. With the exception of a few studies such as those by BRONTË-STEWART *et al.* [1960], KOKERNOT *et al.* [1965], HEINZ [1962], KAMINER and LUTZ [1960] and WYNDHAM and co-workers [WYNDHAM and MORRISON, 1956, 1958; WYNDHAM *et al.*, 1964a, b; WARD *et al.*, 1960], as well as the notable papers in which TOBIAS [1955a, b; 1956a, b; 1960, 1966] consistently related anthropological findings to medical and evolutionary probabilities, little which had appeared provided definite genetic information which could be scrutinized for its bearing on health. Gross human morphology, dependent in the main either on polygenic traits or on complex and ill-understood interactions of inherited and environmental factors, has a connection with health which, though immediately apparent, is difficult to analyze in detail. The proliferation of polymorphisms since that time has admittedly not invariably been revealing on a biomedical level, but it has permitted the assembly of a mass of easily defined data, some of which have already proved to be relevant to health status and much of which may well in the future turn out to be so.

Chapter 3. The Medical Relevance of the Genetic Polymorphisms

Certain genetic polymorphisms have been acknowledged to be medically important since the time of their first discovery. Indeed, it was in a clinical situation, blood transfusion, that many of them were discovered. Others have not yet been shown to have any clinical relevance; yet others present multiple allelism in which one or more alleles are associated with clinical conditions and the rest have no obvious effect on health. It has been established that some genotypes are at an advantage under certain ecological conditions, but not under others, and that a polymorphism which is undoubtedly beneficial in the heterozygous state may be extremely harmful in the homozygous. There are also recognizable situations in which interactions between the effects of two systems, or between gene products and their environmental analogues, may bear significantly on the clinical status of individuals.

The Sensory Polymorphisms

The most immediate reactions between the environment and the polymorphisms might be expected to exist in those polymorphisms which are directly concerned with perception of the environment. Of these, only two have been tested in hunter-gatherer populations in Southern Africa.

Colour Blindness

Post [1962] has reviewed the distribution of defective colour vision in the various populations of the world. He found it to be rarest in groups which either are or have until recently been hunter-gatherers, the Australian Aborigines and American Indians, and in the inhabitants of Fiji, who were presumably largely dependent on fishing. The populations with the highest frequencies were those of Western Europe and certain Far Eastern peoples. He considers that colour blindness must be a handicap in hunting and gathering and tend to be selected against. Since selection would operate most strongly against the hemizygous hunting male and homozygous female, and

Table VI. Colour-blindness among hunter-gatherers

Population	Males		Females		Reference
	n	number affected	n	number affected	
San					
Northern	12	1	11	0	Tobias [1966]
Central	41	0	42	2	Tobias [1966]
Southern	22	0	30	0	Tobias [1966]
Kung	32	1	–	–	Jenkins [1968a]
Southern and Central	56	0	–	–	Jenkins [1968a]
Unspecified	90	2	84	1	Tobias [1972]
Khoi					
Topnaar, Kuiseb	19	1	–	–	Jenkins and Brain [1967]
Negro					
'Kwaai River Hybrids'	19	1	–	–	Jenkins [1968a]

not at all against the majority of heterozygous gathering females, it would probably be a slow process and vary according to the relative importance of the two methods of food procurement. Post's complementary claim that relaxation of selective pressures would lead to an increased frequency in culturally more advanced communities is, however, as Ford [1965] has pointed out, erroneous. This could only happen if the rate of mutation to the condition were unusually high. It seems more likely that positive selection, involving advantages of which we are ignorant, had led to the trend. The medical implications of the polymorphism to hunter-gatherers would, of course, involve not only the procurement of nutrition but the capacity to become aware of dangerous predators.

The frequencies of colour blindness, an X-linked trait, are shown in table VI for all the hunter-gathering peoples of Southern Africa for which figures are available. It will be noted that the figures given by Tobias's [1966] review show frequencies much larger than those in the same author's [1972] paper on Southern Africa. It seems likely that the earlier figures are mistaken, due probably to a sampling error. All other studies show the San, and the Khoi, to have frequencies which accord very well with expectations on Post's hypothesis.

Phenylthiocarbamide (PTC) Tasting Ability and Goitre

Harris *et al.* [1949] found that 41% of 134 persons with nodular goitre were unable to taste PTC, while the recessively inherited inability was only found in 31% of 541 normal persons and 31% of 218 persons with toxic diffuse goitre. KITCHIN *et al.* [1959] confirmed these findings for persons with nodular goitre but found significantly fewer, 15% of 133 tested, in the group with toxic diffuse goitre. When their figures for the nodular goitre group were broken down according to sex, 79 out of 218 females, 36.2%, were non-tasters, as were 18 out of 28, or 66.3%, of the males. This observation led them to the conclusion that the taster genotype might be important in determining the type of thyroid disease a person might develop, and that the importance of the genotype was twice as great in males as in females.

Only three Southern African hunter-gatherer populations have been tested for this polymorphism so far. JENKINS [1965] found 6 non-tasters among 49 male Central San. All of the 36 females he tested were able to taste PTC. In 1967, JENKINS and BRAIN [1967] tested 29 Kuiseb Topnaar and found 6 non-tasters among them, 4 males and 2 females. Six Dama, one of whom was a non-taster, were tested at the same time. There were only two female non-tasters among the 38 Kgalagadi (24 males and 14 females) who have been tested [JENKINS, 1965].

The low phenotypic incidence of inability to taste the substance would probably make the investigation of the polymorphism less informative among Southern African hunter-gatherers than among many other populations. Some cases of enlargement of the thyroid have been found among the San, but they show no significant association with inability to taste PTC [JENKINS, 1972]. On the other hand, there is a distinct difference between the sexes in this polymorphism. Females have a higher PTC-tasting threshold and goitre is distinctly commoner in females than in males. The San show a significantly higher frequency of non-tasters among the males ($\chi^2_{[1]} = 4.60$) while the excess among the female Kgalagadi just escapes significance at the 5% level ($\chi^2_{[1]} = 3.60$). It is difficult to account for these opposing trends, as the latter is in the opposite direction to that usually found in hunter-gatherers [JENKINS, 1972]. Certain vegetable goitrogens are thiocarbamides [WILLIAMS and BAKKE, 1962], and it could be suggested that consumption of such vegetables despite their bitter taste might be responsible for an association between the polymorphism and the disease. It may be that an ability to reject such goitrogens is of selective value in hunter-gatherer populations, and could account for the San frequencies. This argument makes it difficult, however, to explain the quite high gene frequencies in the three other populations tested. The flora used as food by the Dama and the Topnaar of the Kuiseb may well differ from that in the Kalahari, but the Kgalagadi share the same biotope as the San. It is perhaps significant that their frequency of the gene is lower than that in the Topnaar or in the pitifully tiny sample of Dama tested, though none of these samples is of sufficient size for comparative selective trends against the inability to taste to be postulated with any degree of certainty.

Thyroid enlargement was found in 6 males and 7 females in a series of 49 male and 31 female San. One of the male cases was a non-taster out of a total of 5 non-tasters in the series. All the female cases were tasters, and there was no significant association between the conditions. The occurrence of goitre could be ascribed to vegetable goitrogens, possibly not thioureas or thiocarbamides but analogous to those responsible for the goitre association with the 'spring flush' described by CLEMENTS and WISHART [1955]. Endemic goitre associated with fluoride excess has been described in settled Kalahari populations [STEYN, 1948], but no dental evidence of excess of fluorides has been found in San [TRUSWELL and HANSEN, 1968b] except for a few instances of mottled teeth in the population which also included the goitrous individuals mentioned above. It is possible, however, that in mild degrees of iodine depletion and the presence of goitrogens in the diet, a slight excess of fluoride may exert a cytotoxic effect on the thyroid [NURSE and WOOD, 1967].

The Metabolic Polymorphisms

Two polymorphisms, variation in which is detected by the administration of test substances to the subjects and subsequent quantitative assessment of the resulting metabolites, and which appear to be inherited in a simple Mendelian fashion, have been investigated in two hunter-gatherer populations in Southern Africa. One has also been tested in a settled Khoi population. The frequencies found for both may represent environmental adaptations.

Lactose Intolerance or Intestinal Lactase Deficiency

Except in comparatively rare cases, hunter-gatherer populations do not possess domesticated cattle. Even cattle-rearing peoples often either do not consume milk or consume it prepared in such a way that its lactose content is converted to lactic acid. The presence of intestinal lactase subsequent to weaning in sufficient quantity for ingested lactose to be converted to, and absorbed as, glucose, is virtually confined to the Caucasoids of North-Western Europe and America and a few pastoral peoples [SIMOONS, 1970]. The fact that a high prevalence of lactose intolerance may vitiate the effectiveness of nutritional programmes in which large quantities of milk powder are distributed to non-Caucasoid peoples has been pointed out by KRETSCHMER [1972]. Milk powder is a cheap and readily available dietary supplement

Table VII. Lactose tolerance and acetylator status

Population	n	Phenotype frequency				Gene frequency	
		lactose		acetylation			
		tolerant	intolerant	rapid	slow	*lactose tolerance*	*slow acetylation*
San							
!Kung, Tsumkwe[17]	40	1	39	–	–	0.013 ± 0.012	
	30	–	–	29	1		0.235 ± 0.077
‡huã:[13]	25	2	23	–	–	0.040 ± 0.028	
	15	–	–	14	1	–	0.258 ± 0.113
Khoi							
Nama adults[18]	18	9	9	–	–	0.293 ± 0.107	–
Nama children[18]	21	4	17	–	–	0.100 ± 0.065	–
Negro							
Dama	5	0	5	–	–	0.000	
Denasena[15]	50	0	50	–	–	0.000	

χ^2 [1] between Nama adults and children = 4.18, 0.05 > p.

widely distributed to the undernourished by the well-meaning. The hunter-gatherers of the Southern African deserts are beginning to make occasional use of trading-stores, and dried and evaporated milk are available to them; this applies in particular to one of the populations investigated and found to be generally intolerant of lactose [JENKINS *et al.*, 1974]. The other [NURSE and JENKINS, 1974] lives in a periodic client/patron relationship with some settled Kgalagadi who have cattle and may be expected to consume both fresh and fermented milk.

The main danger of the administration of lactose to intolerant persons is that diarrhoea in infants and children may be provoked or exacerbated. It is important that the lactase status of a population should be investigated before milk or milk powder is introduced as a foodstuff, not in order that the introduction should be stopped but rather that the lactose should be rendered inoffensive by fermentation. The figures for the !Kung of Tsumkwe and the ‡huã: of south-eastern central Botswana are given in table VII. The results of an investigation of the Nama are included, despite the fact that the sample studied represented a settled urban community, mainly to show that it is possible that some individuals of this community, like certain of the Yoruba mentioned by KRETSCHMER [1972], may become tolerant to lactose through induction of the enzyme by continuing milk consumption. There were significantly more tolerant adults than children. That there were any tolerant San at all is of particular interest, in view of the suggestion by SIMOONS [1970] that this dominantly inherited variant has reached its high local frequencies elsewhere on account of the advantage it confers in a culture which makes use of dairy products. It would seem to suggest either that mutation to tolerance has occurred independently in two widely separated hunter-gatherer communities, or that the San may be yet another people which has reverted to hunting and gathering following a period of pastoralism or settlement. It is naturally also possible that the gene has been introduced by admixture.

Even more puzzling results have, in fact, been found in a dairying community where other gene marker studies have established probable admixture proportions of 50% Caucasoid and 50% Nama Khoi. Only 20 adult Basters of Rehoboth have so far been tested, but of these 20 only 7 were lactose-tolerant. This is not significantly different from the figure for Nama adults ($\chi^2_{[1]} = 0.85$) but it is from BAYLESS and ROSENSWEIG's [1966] figure for a North American Caucasoid sample of the same size ($\chi^2_{[1]} = 12.91$). Considering the extensive use made of unfermented milk by the Basters one would have expected selective forces to have inclined the proportion of those tolerant towards the Caucasoid rather than the Khoi frequency. If the locus is subject to selection, it might be some factor other than milk consumption which is principally involved; possibly selection could be acting more strongly in a desert environment on an unidentified locus in linkage disequilibrium with that for lactase than on the ability to metabolize milk sugar. More work is needed in this field.

Acetylator Status

With the penetration of other peoples into their fastnesses, the hunter-gatherer group in Southern Africa are steadily becoming exposed to a variety of infectious diseases against which their inherited or acquired resistance can be expected to be low. Tuberculosis, in particular, afflicts certain of them seriously and often; and the antituberculous agent most frequently prescribed for those who do present for treatment is isonicotinyl hydrazide (isoniazid). The effectiveness of the treatment naturally depends on the rapidity with which isoniazid is metabolized, and it has been shown that there is a polymorphism of liver acetyl transferase which governs this [EVANS, 1962]. If the dose administered is metabolized too rapidly, the efficacy of the drug is reduced; if too slowly, the accumulation of the drug may lead to peripheral neuritis due to competitive inhibition of the action of pyridoxine. Tests carried out on the !Kung of Tsumkwe [JENKINS *et al.*, 1974] and the ǂhuã: have shown a very low frequency of the recessive homozygote for slow acetylation, coupled with a rapidity of acetylation in excess of that found in other populations. The tests were performed only on the urine, whereas EVANS [1969] has shown that serum estimations give better phenotypic discrimination. Using the same test schedules as he, and regarding the percentage acetylation 6 h after administration of the test drug as having been rapid if above 62.5%, it appears that 18 of his 37 Caucasoid rapid acetylators had metabolized 85% or more of the drug. In the !Kung the figure was 23 out of 30, and in the ‡huã: 11 out of 14. It is possible that what is responsible here is not so much a genetically controlled exceptional rapidity of acetylation as a relative excess of drug circulating unbound to albumen and consequently more available for quick acetylation [BUCHANAN, personal commun., 1974]. The serum albumen level is relatively low in the San [TOBIAS, 1966; BRONTË-STEWART *et al.*, 1963] and this would lend credence to this hypothesis. Whatever the explanation, both the rapid elimination of the drug and the presence of the gene for slow acetylation in the San would seem to indicate that an assessment of acetylator status is advisable prior to deciding the optimum dosage in each case of tuberculosis. The figures for the two populations are shown in table VII.

Liver acetyl transferase is involved in the metabolism of other drugs than isoniazid, though none of these is likely to be used as often in the treatment of hunter-gatherer patients. The function of the enzyme in non-therapeutic situations is not known for certain, but it probably helps in the detoxification of a variety of ingested substances. The low frequency of slow acetylation in the San is similar to that of another hunter-gatherer population, the Canadian Eskimo [ARMSTRONG and PEART, 1960], and the differences in type of foodstuffs between these two peoples might suggest either that the range of efficacy of the enzyme must be very wide, or that similarities yet to be identified between the ways of life exist, for this resemblance to be selectively explicable. It may, of course, simply be due to random drift.

Polymorphisms of the Cell Surface

Certain genetic polymorphisms were first shown to exist by the demonstration of immune reactions involving antigens on the cell surface. Some of these polymorphisms were early recognized to be of medical importance; for others, disease associations ostensibly only remotely related to their immunological particularities have only been discovered later. All the clinically relevant polymorphisms of this class are investigated by the reactions of antibodies of known specificity with surface antigens of cell membranes. The antigens which occur on non-nucleated cells, the blood group antigens, are found also on nucleated cells, but there are two or more sets which are absent from non-nucleated cells such as erythrocytes.

The Tissue Antigen Systems

Except in the possible context of specific disease associations, the medical applications of these systems to the Southern African hunter-gatherers seems at present to be remote. It is unlikely that tissue transplantation will soon become a part of their way of life. On the other hand, the association of certain tissue specificities with auto-immune diseases is now a recognized phenomenon, and one whose diminished relevance here is due in the main to the paucity of our information about auto-immune disease in the populations we are discussing. The data presented in tables VIIIa and b are taken from NURSE *et al.* [1975], and represent a reworking of the data originally presented

Table VIIIa. The HLA polymorphism: haplotype frequencies

Haplotype		Frequencies			
first series	second series	San		Khoi	
		Northern !Kung (n = 81)	Tsumkwe !Kung (= 123)	Hei//om (n = 60)	Nama (n = 106)
A1	Bw17	0.030	0.001	0.015	0.016
A2	B7	0.060	0.000	0.029	0.002
A2	B8	0.018	0.048	0.000	0.011
A2	B12	0.000	0.029	0.025	0.016
A3	Bw40	0.050	0.007	0.010	0.010
A3	Bw15	0.005	0.000	0.003	0.020
Aw23	Bw14	0.000	0.000		0.019
Aw23	Bw17	0.054	0.003	0.003	0.020
Aw24	B7	0.004	0.025	0.009	0.022
Aw25	Bw35	0.014	0.000	0.000	0.003
A28	B8	0.003	0.026	0.005	0.000
A28	Bw35	0.000	0.002	0.000	0.022
A29	B18	0.010	0.003	0.013	0.023
Aw30	B5	0.007	0.003	0.022	0.019
Aw30	B12	0.044	0.020	0.000	0.008
Aw32	B8		0.006	0.028	0.000
Aw32	B14		0.032		0.000
Aw33	Bw22		0.011	0.000	0.000
BK(Aw43)	B7		0.020		0.012
BK(Aw43)	B12		0.000		0.036

Adapted from NURSE *et al.* [1975]. Since the number of haplotypes is very large, only those giving significant Δ-associations (0.05 > p) in one or more of the populations are shown here. Blanks represent the absence from the population of one of the components of a haplotype.

Table VIIIb. The HLA polymorphism: gene frequencies

Gene	Frequencies			
	San		Khoi	
	Northern !Kung (n = 81)	Tsumkwe !Kung (n = 123)	Hei//om (n = 60)	Nama (n = 106)
First (HLA) locus				
A1	0.05	0.01	0.05	0.06
A2	0.16	0.19	0.15	0.13
A3	0.08	0.20	0.05	0.07
A9(Aw23+Aw24)	0.13	0.15	0.17	0.14
A10(Aw25+Aw26)	0.07	0.03	0.02	0.14
A28	0.05	0.07	0.08	0.09
Aw19: A29	0.01	0.01	0.06	0.07
Aw19: Aw30	0.26	0.21	0.14	0.09
Aw19: Aw31+Aw32	0.01	0.05	0.16	0.06
Aw19: Aw33	0.09	0.03	0.07	0.04
BK(Aw43)	0.00	0.05	0.00	0.09
Blank	0.07	0.00	0.03	0.03
Second (four) locus				
B5	0.09	0.03	0.09	0.06
B7	0.19	0.09	0.11	0.14
B8	0.04	0.13	0.04	0.03
B12	0.06	0.06	0.07	0.14
B13	0.02	0.00	0.02	0.02
Bw15+Bw35	0.05	0.05	0.12	0.13
Bw40	0.12	0.10	0.12	0.07
B14	0.01	0.04	0.00	0.07
Bw16	0.00	0.00	0.03	0.02
Bw17	0.24	0.37	0.22	0.13
B18	0.04	0.02	0.06	0.07
Bw21+Bw22	0.01	0.03	0.02	0.02
B27	0.00	0.00	0.01	0.03
Blank	0.12	0.08	0.11	0.09

Adapted from NURSE *et al.* [1975]. W21 is found only in the Northern !Kung, in whom W22 does not occur.

in BOTHA *et al.* [1973]. They constitute all the material presently available about the tissue antigen systems in these populations; the single sample of settled Khoi Nama from Keetmanshoop and Berseba is included to emphasize the essential similarity of the Khoi with the San. Indeed, there seems to be an overall 'Southern African' HLA pattern, consisting of high frequencies of W30 in the first, and W17 in the second, segregant series, absence of HLA-A11 and low frequencies of HLA-A1; this agrees broadly with the patterns detected in settled Southern African Negroes by BRAIN and HAMMOND

[1973] and FESTENSTEIN *et al.* [1973]. The 'BK' antigen (HLA-Aw43) mentioned is first described by NURSE *et al.* [1975]. It is a member of the first segregant series and appears to 'bridge' HLA-A10 and W29.

The Red Cell Antigens and Blood Transfusion

The Kell and Duffy Systems

One type of tissue transplantation to which individual hunter-gatherers of Southern Africa are periodically exposed as medical attention becomes more readily available to them is blood transfusion. It has been shown that if the ABO antigens and rhesus D are disregarded, the comparative rarity of other strong antigens on the erythrocytes of the San makes them slightly less hazardous as donors and marginally more in danger as recipients in whom antibody production may be stimulated [NURSE and JENKINS, 1973a]. In fact, the Khoi and the Negroes also either have low frequencies of the antigenically more powerful blood group phenotypes, relative to Caucasoids and Mongoloids, or else have such high frequencies that individuals lacking the antigen and consequently liable to sensitization are rare not often found. The most potent antigens in the rhesus system are D, c, E, e and C, in that order [GIBLETT, 1961]; the two former and the fourth are almost universal in all San and Khoi populations, but the Dama have a curiously low frequency of D. There is rather more C among the Khoi and more E among the Dama, while among the San C frequencies increase from south to north and E from west to east (tables XIa, b).

The Kell antigen K and the Duffy antigen Fy(a) are the only two remaining ones of sufficient antigenic potency to be at all likely to be responsible for transfusion reactions. The claim by ZOUTENDYK *et al.* [1953] that the frequency of K among the San was even higher than among Caucasoids has not been substantiated by later work; it is rare in or absent from all the populations considered here. The 2 Kell positives among the 147 Nharo give a gene frequency of 0.007, and the 7 out of 165 //au//en give 0.021. One out of 58 Kuiseb Topnaar was positive for K, and the resulting gene frequency is 0.009. The remaining populations did not contain a single positive. On the other hand, Fy(a) occurs in the Khoisan at high frequencies while Negroes often lack any Duffy antigen detectable with the sera available. MILLER *et al.* [1975] have shown that the Fy(a) and Fy(b) antigens act as cell surface receptors facilitating invasion by the simian malaria parasite *P. knowlesii*. They suggest that the lack of these antigens by Negroes in West Africa and

Table IX. Duffy phenotypes and gene frequencies

Population	n		Phenotypes				Gene frequencies			χ²
			Fy(a+b–)	Fy(a+b+)	Fy(a–b+)	Fy(a–b–)	*Fy*ᵃ	*Fy*ᵇ	*Fy*	
San										
G!aokx'ate[10]	33	obs.	5	16	12	0	0.394	0.606	0.000	0.
		exp.	5.1	15.8	12.1	0				
!Xõ[16]	51	obs.	9	22	17	3	0.348	0.466	0.186	4.
		exp.	12.8	16.5	19.9	1.8				
ǂhuã:[13]	36	obs.	7	9	14	6	0.240	0.370	0.390	1.
		exp.	8.8	6.4	15.3	5.5				
G/wi[7]	94		58		36		0.381	0.619		
G//ana[7]	50		24		26		0.279	0.721		
Nharo[6]	147		70		77		0.276	0.724		
//au//en[6]	185		106		76		0.347	0.654		
!Kung, Dobe[6]	385		174		213		0.260	0.740		
!Kung, /ai/ai[6]	64		32		32		0.293	0.707		
!Kung, /du/da[6]	54		28		26		0.307	0.693		
!Kung, Tsumkwe[6]	279		151		128		0.323	0.677		
!Kung, G!ãg!ai[10]	36	obs.	8	12	14	2	0.334	0.447	0.219	0.
		exp.	9.3	10.7	14.3	1.7				
Khoi										
Topnaar, Kuiseb[9]	13		11		2		0.608	0.392		
Topnaar, Sesfontein[6]	42		12		30		0.155	0.845		
Hei//om[10]	96		22		74		0.122	0.878		
Negro										
Dama[12]	90	obs.	3	2	7	78	0.046	0.065	0.889	8.
		exp.	7.6	0.5	10.8	71.1				
Kwengo[14]	35	obs.	2	0	6	27	0.029	0.086	0.885	0.
		exp.	1.8	0.2	5.6	27.4				
Denasena[15]	77	obs.	14	0	5	60	0.093	0.032	0.875	0.
		exp.	13.5	0.5	4.5	60.5				

their rarity in the rest of the continent may explain the almost complete absence of *P. vivax* infestation except in those areas where the antigens occur. The only other known medical significance of the Kell and Duffy systems is in the fields of haemolytic disease of the newborn and blood transfusion. The results of tests on Southern African hunter-gatherer populations for variation in the Duffy system are shown in table IX. The ABO and rhesus systems, whose clinical importance is greater, are treated separately.

The ABO System

The importance of ABO compatibility in blood transfusion is too familiar to need much discussion. The presence of weak A groups in high frequencies in many Southern African populations can, however, present particular local problems. As is well known, individuals of a weak A group can possess anti-A_1 in the serum, and the administration of group A_1 blood to them can be dangerous. JENKINS [1974] has pointed out how common the A_{bantu} blood group is in the Khoisan, and that under less than ideal circumstances this group can be mistaken for O. In a recipient this would be of little moment, but the administration of A_{bantu} donor blood to an O recipient is probably not a safe procedure. It can be seen from table Xa that A_2 and A_{bantu} are the only A groups in the ‡huã:, and that both are common in most San populations; though not found in the small samples of Khoi hunter-gatherers, apart from the Hei//om, they do occur in settled Khoi populations. The A_2 reported among the Dama by KNUSSMANN [1969] was probably $A_{intermediate}$ [NURSE *et al.*, 1976], which has been pooled with A_1 in all the series set out here. A_2, but not A_{bantu}, was found in the Kwengo, and both occur in the Denasena, though the frequency of A_{bantu} is extremely low (table Xb).

The A_{bantu} phenotype was first characterized by BRAIN [1966] and thus named because he believed it to be a 'Bantu' (Negro) characteristic. JENKINS [1974] has shown, however, that it is much commoner in the San and Khoi than in the Negro tribes of Southern Africa and, because of its virtual

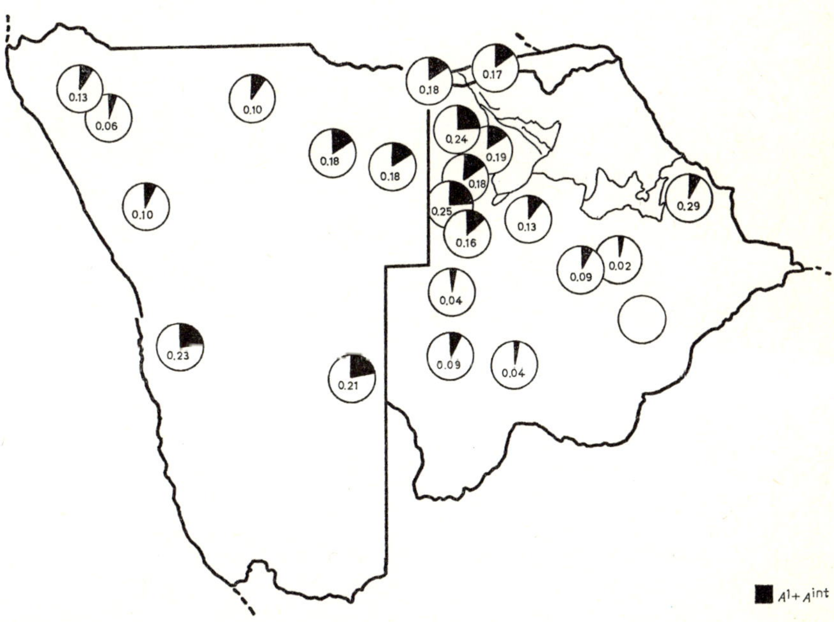

Fig. 3. The distribution of the stronger variants of A in the ABO blood group system.

Table Xa. The ABO blood group phenotypes and gene frequencies in the San

Population	n		Phenotypes								Gene frequencies					χ^{2a}	d.f.
			A_2+A_{int}	A_2	A_{bantu}	$A_1B+A_{int}B$	A_2B	$A_{bantu}B$	B	O	A^1+A^{int}	A_2	A^{bantu}	B	O		
G!aokx'ate[10]	33	obs.	12	3	5	0	0	0	1	12	0.206	0.061	0.115	0.015	0.603	0.66	1
		exp.	12.0	3.0	5.0	0.2	0.1	0.1	0.6	12.0							
Southern, mainly !Xõ[6]	72	obs.	12	7	2	0	1	0	4	46	0.087	0.063	0.017	0.035	0.798	0.11	1
		exp.	11.6	7.7	1.9	0.4	0.3	0.1	4.2	45.9							
!Xõ[16]	51	obs.	3	7	2	0	0	2	1	36	0.040	0.099	0.036	0.037	0.788	5.24	1
		exp.	3.8	8.8	3.0	0.2	0.4	0.1	3.0	31.7							
ǂhuã[13]	36	obs.	0	2	3	0	0	0	3	28	0	0.029	0.046	0.043	0.882	0.21	1
		exp.	0	2.0	3.0	0	0.1	0.1	2.8	28.0							
G/wi[7]	94	obs.	16	16	6	0	1	0	3	52	0.091	0.102	0.042	0.021	0.744	0.00	1
		exp.	16.0	16.0	6.0	0.2	0.4	0.2	3.0	52.0							
G//ana[7]	50	obs.	2	1	7	1	0	0	2	37	0.021	0.011	0.078	0.030	0.860	1.81	1
		exp.	2.0	1.0	7.0	0.1	0.0	0.2	2.6	37.0							
Nharo[6]	149	obs.	39	4	4	0	1	0	3	98	0.141	0.020	0.016	0.013	0.809	0.23	1
		exp.	38.5	4.9	3.9	0.6	0.1	0.1	3.3	97.7							
//au//en[6]	264	obs.	79	2	5	0	1	0	16	161	0.163	0.007	0.011	0.033	0.785	5.00	2
		exp.	76.4	2.9	4.8	2.8	0.1	0.2	13.9	162.8							
!Kung[8]	72	obs.	22	13	4	1	1	0	4	27	0.175	0.128	0.041	0.043	0.614	0.03	2
		exp.	21.9	13.2	3.8	1.1	0.8	0.3	3.9	27.1							
!Kung, Northern[6]	104	obs.	35	13	2	0	0	0	0	54	0.186	0.081	0.013	0	0.721	0.00	1
		exp.	35.0	13.0	2.0	0	0	0	0	54.0							
!Kung, Ngami[6]	156	obs.	36	22	9	1	2	0	10	76	0.127	0.093	0.038	0.043	0.700	1.34	3
		exp.	35.4	22.8	8.5	1.7	1.2	0.3	9.6	76.3							
!Kung, Dobe[6]	436	obs.	181	10	25	2	2	0	13	203	0.239	0.018	0.040	0.020	0.684	2.46	2
		exp.	179.2	11.7	24.3	4.1	0.3	0.7	11.9	203.8							
!Kung, /ai/ai[6]	65	obs.	28	4	0	0	0	0	2	31	0.247	0.042	0	0.016	0.696	0.83	2
		exp.	27.6	3.9	0	0.5	0.1	0	1.4	31.5							
!Kung, du/da[6]	102	obs.	33	1	4	0	0	0	2	62	0.178	0.006	0.024	0.009	0.782	0.20	1
		exp.	32.7	0.9	3.9	0.4	0.0	0.1	1.6	62.4							
!Kung, Tsumkwe[6]	279	obs.	91	11	23	1	0	0	12	141	0.182	0.025	0.054	0.024	0.716	2.52	2
		exp.	89.7	10.7	22.4	2.4	0.3	0.7	9.6	143.1							
!Kung, G!ãg!ai[10]	36	obs.	11	1	6	0	1	0	2	15	0.176	0.018	0.118	0.042	0.646	0.00	1
		exp.	11.0	1.0	6.0	0.5	0.1	0.4	2.0	15.0							

[a] The AB phenotypes have been pooled for calculation of χ^2.

Table Xb. The ABO blood group phenotypes and gene frequencies in Khoi and Negroes

Population	n		Phenotypes								Gene frequencies					χ^{2a}	d.f.
			A_1+A_{int}	A_2	A_{bantu}	$A_1B+A_{int}B$	A_2B	$A_{bantu}B$	B	O	A^1+A^{int}	A^2	A^{bantu}	B	O		
Khoi																	
Topnaar, Kuiseb[9]	58	obs.	15	0	0	9	0	0	14	20	0.229	0.000	0.000	0.218	0.553	2.93	1
		exp.	17.7	0	0	5.8	0	0	16.7	17.7							
Topnaar, Sesfontein[6]	42	obs.	9	0	0	1	2	0	14	16	0.129	0.028	0.000	0.228	0.615	1.12	1
		exp.	7.6	1.5	0	2.5	0.5	0	14.0	15.9							
Hei//om[10]	96	obs.	17	4	3	0	1	0	10	61	0.098	0.025	0.019	0.059	0.797	0.03	1
		exp.	16.7	4.0	2.9	1.1	0.3	0.2	9.4	61.0							
Negro																	
Dama[11]	448	obs.	38	5	0	14	4	0	177	210	0.061	0.006	0.000	0.249	0.685	0.35	1
		exp.	39.4	3.7	0	13.6	1.3	0	180.6	210.2							
Dama[12]	119	obs.	16	0	0	9	0	0	47	47	0.099	0.000	0.000	0.272	0.629	1.21	1
		exp.	16.0	0	0	6.4	0	0	49.5	47.1							
Kwengo[14]	35	obs.	12	3	0	0	0	0	10	10	0.169	0.075	0.000	0.221	0.535	5.54	2
		exp.	8.2	3.0	0	2.6	1.2	0	10.0	10.0							
Denasena[15]	79	obs.	11	5	1	2	1	2	16	41	0.085	0.042	0.009	0.143	0.721	1.41	1
		exp.	10.9	4.9	0.9	1.9	1.0	0.2	18.1	41.0							

[a] The AB phenotypes have been pooled for calculation of χ^2.

absence in Negro populations to the north, has postulated that it is primarily a Khoisan character which has only secondarily been acquired by the Negroes as they migrated southwards; other genes similarly acquired are $Gm^{1,13}$, Fy^{a} and acid phosphatase P^{r} (chapter 6).

Haemolytic disease of the newborn due to feto-maternal ABO incompatibility is likely to be relatively more important in peoples in whom the frequency of rhesus negativity is low, and in fact it is the commonest type of the disease encountered in South African Negroes [ZOUTENDYK, 1962]. ZOUTENDYK was under the impression that the disease was more common and more severe when the offending antigen on the baby's red cells was B, but JENKINS [1972] has shown that though A_1 appears to be a slightly more potent cause there is in fact no consistent significant difference. Though no clinically established cases of the disease have been reported among Southern African Khoisan hunter-gatherers, it is worth pointing out that B is not very common in the San or the Hei//om, and that the frequency of A_1 tends to

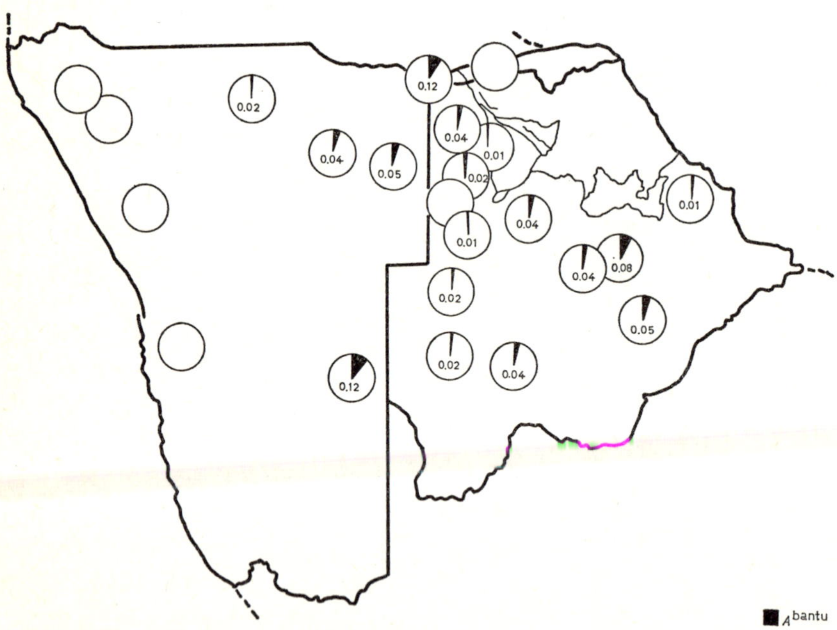

Fig. 4. The distribution of the weak A allele A^{bantu} in the ABO system. It will be seen that frequencies are highest in the San populations and tend to be low or non-existent in the Negro and Khoi populations. In fact, settled populations of these two races tend to have higher frequencies of the gene, suggesting a large San contribution to them.

fall from north to south. The Khoi, on the other hand, in common with the Dama, Denasena and Kwengo Negroes, have high frequencies of B, moderate to high frequencies of A_1, and comparatively low frequencies of the weak A groups. It has been pointed out by SCHELLONG [1964] that the potency of the ABO antigens before and shortly after birth is not as high as in the adult, and that this could represent a protective mechanism.

TOBIAS [1966] has suggested that the very high frequency of B among the Khoi may be explicable on the contention of VOGEL *et al.* [1960] that group B individuals are better able to resist smallpox. Large-scale smallpox epidemics ravaged the Cape area during the 18th century, and the possession of B could have represented a selective advantage and led to the survival of proportionately more persons of that group. It is possible that the more remote San populations would have escaped the epidemics, but it would seem surprising if the then equally remote Dama, Denasena and Kwengo should nevertheless have been afflicted.

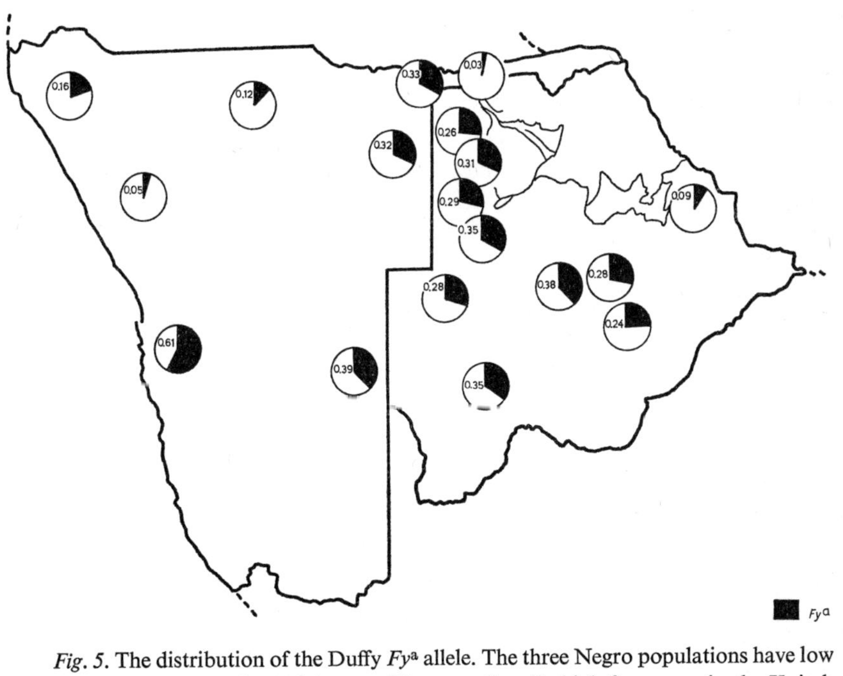

Fig. 5. The distribution of the Duffy *Fy*ª allele. The three Negro populations have low frequencies, and the Khoisan high ones. The exceptionally high frequency in the Kuiseb Khoi may be due in part to Caucasoid admixture.

The Rhesus System

As can be seen from the data in tables XIa and b the San and the Khoi have low frequencies of rhesus negativity, except in the cases of !Kung reported by JENKINS *et al.* [1968] and JENKINS [1972]. The former came from Xoshi and Xangwa in north-western Botswana, and the latter from Dobe in the same region, and probably represent much the same geographical and mating population. The Dama by contrast have not only a comparatively high frequency of *r* for an African population but also possess two other alleles, *r′* and *r″*, which do not produce D substance [KNUSSMANN, 1969]. KNUSSMANN does not mention whether he found any D^u individuals and, if so, whether they were accounted rhesus positive or negative. Even when a Dama sample is sorted to exclude related individuals, and the D^u antigen is counted as D, rhesus negativity remains much more common than it is in the Khoisan, though in absolute figures it becomes comparable with other Negro populations [NURSE *et al.*, 1976]. The Denasena *r* frequency is in the same range, but this population does not appear to have *r′* or *r″*. The only rhesus-negative allele other than *r* probably present in a Khoisan population is *r′* in one sample of !Kung.

These findings become of obvious significance when one considers the possible occurrence of haemolytic disease of the newborn due to rhesus incompatibility. We have been unable to find any account of this disease in any of the hunter-gatherer peoples, even the Dama, but it seems very unlikely that it does not occur in the latter and the Denasena. The presence of *r′* and *r″* could also be expected to be of importance in blood transfusion situations; this is particularly relevant, again, to the Dama, who have adapted very readily to urban life and are to be found in Windhoek in great numbers. In transfusions the D^u antigen also needs to be taken into account.

The frequency of R^0 is very high in the Khoisan; two small samples those of the !Xõ of western Botswana and the G!ãg!ai !Kung of the Kavango area, showed no evidence of possessing any other allele. Comparatively high frequencies of R^1 have been found in the Khoi and the northern San, becoming lower to the south; the R^2 frequencies show a less regular cline, and are generally low in the San except in the G//ana [JENKINS *et al.*, 1975] and, it seems, the ‡huã:. They are moderate in the Khoi and Negroes. An apparent excess of R^2 homozygotes in the Denasena can be accounted for by the presence of an apparent *cD*-allele in fairly high frequency. Homozygotes for this allele have been found in the population, and are in process of being investigated. The consequent adjustment of the frequencies shown in table XIb

Table XIa. Rhesus blood group phenotypes and gene frequencies in the San

Population	n		Phenotypes									Gene frequencies					χ^2	d.f.
			ccDee	CcDee	ccDEe	CcDEe	CCDee	ccDEE	ccdee	Ccdee	CCdee	R⁰	R^1	R^2	r	r'		
G!aokx'ate[10]	33	obs.	27	6	0	0	0	0	0	0	0	0.909	0.091	0.000	0.000	0.000	0.37	1
		exp.	27.3	5.4	0	0	0.3	0	0	0	0							
Southern, mainly !Xõ[6]	72	obs.	68	2	1	0	0	0	1	0	0	0.861	0.014	0.007	0.118	0.000	0.00	1
		exp.	68.0	2.0	1.0	0	0	0	1.0	0	0							
!Xõ[16]	51	obs.	51	0	0	0	0	0	0	0	0	1.000	0.000	0.000	0.000	0.000	–	–
		exp.	51.0	0	0	0	0	0	0	0	0							
ǂhuã[13]	36	obs.	26	2	7	1	0	0	0	0	0	0.847	0.042	0.111	0.000	0.000	2.24	2
		exp.	25.8	2.6	6.8	0.3	0.1	0.4	0	0	0							
G/wi[7]	94	obs.	89	2	1	0	1	1	0	0	0	0.963	0.021	0.016	0.000	0.000	0.58[a]	1
		exp.	87.2	3.8	2.9	0.1	0.0	0.0	0	0	0							
G//ana[7]	50	obs.	41	1	8	0	0	0	0	0	0	0.865	0.010	0.125	0.000	0.000	1.98	1
		exp.	37.4	0.9	10.8	0.1	0.0	0.8	0	0	0							
Nharo[6]	147	obs.	139	5	2	0	0	0	1	0	0	0.901	0.017	0.007	0.075	0.000	3.06	1
		exp.	138.2	4.9	1.9	0.0	0.1	0.0	0.8	0	0							
//au//en[6]	210	obs.	194	9	6	0	0	0	1	0	0	0.895	0.021	0.014	0.069	0.000	0.28	1
		exp.	194.3	8.7	5.8	0.1	0.1	0.0	1.0	0	0							
!Kung[8]	71	obs.	44	20	0	0	5	0	2	0	0	0.641	0.186	0.000	0.159	0.014	0.60	1
		exp.	43.6	21.1	0	0	4.1	0	1.8	0.3	0.0							
!Kung, Northern[6]	104	obs.	76	21	0	0	6	0	1	0	0	0.745	0.159	0.000	0.096	0.000	6.17	2
		exp.	72.7	27.8	0	0	2.6	0	1.0	0	0							
!Kung, Ngami[6]	157	obs	125	27	0	0	5	0	0	0	0	0.882	0.118	0.000	0.000	0.000	4.49	1
		exp.	122.1	32.6	0	0	2.2	0	0	0	0							
!Kung, Dobe[6]	383	obs.	337	35	2	0	0	0	9	0	0	0.798	0.046	0.003	0.154	0.000	0.99	1
		exp.	337.9	33.3	1.9	0.1	0.8	0.0	9.0	0	0							
!Kung, /ai/ai[6]	63	obs.	52	8	1	0	0	0	2	0	0	0.929	0.064	0.008	0.000	0.000	0.34	2
		exp.	52.4	7.4	0.8	0.1	0.3	0.0	1.9	0	0							
!Kung, /du/da[6]	102	obs.	95	7	0	0	0	0	0	0	0	0.966	0.034	0.000	0.000	0.000	0.13	1
		exp.	95.1	6.8	0	0	0.1	0	0	0	0							
!Kung, Tsumkwe[6]	279	obs.	258	19	1	0	0	0	1	0	0	0.904	0.035	0.002	0.060	0.000	0.00	1
		exp.	258.0	19.0	1.0	0.0	0	0.0	1.0	0	0							
!Kung, G!ãg!ai[10]	36	obs.	36	0	0	0	0	0	0	0	0	1.000	0.000	0.000	0.000	0.000	–	–
		exp.	36.0	0	0	0	0	0	0	0	0	0.182	0.025	0.054	0.024	0.716	2.52	2

[a] Derived by pooling apparent homozygotes for R^1 and R^2 with heterozygotes (see text).

Table XIb. Rhesus blood group phenotypes and gene frequencies in Khoi and Negroes

Population	n		Phenotypes												Gene frequencies						χ^2	d.f.
			ccDee	CcDee	ccDEe	CcDEe	CCDee	ccDEE	ccdee	Ccdee	ccdEe	CCdee	CcdEe	ccdEE	R⁰	R^1	R^2	r	r'	r''		
Topnaar, Kuiseb[9]	58	obs.	39	12	4	3	0	0	0	0	0	0	0	0	0.810	0.129	0.060	0.000	0.000	0.000	6.55	3
		exp.	38.1	12.2	5.7	0.9	1.0	0.2	0	0	0	0	0	0								
Topnaar, Sesfontein[6]	42	obs.	28	7	3	2	2	0	0	0	0	0	0	0	0.786	0.155	0.060	0.000	0.000	0.000	4.76	2
		exp.	25.9	10.2	4.0	0.8	1.0	0.2	0	0	0	0	0	0								
Hei//om[10]	96	obs.	72	15	4	2	2	0	1	0	0	.	0	0	0.764	0.103	0.038	0.095	0.000	0.000	3.94	2
		exp.	70.0	17.0	6.2	0.7	1.0	0.1	0.9	0	0	0	0	0								
Negro																						
Dama[11]	448	obs.	[illegible]7	35	81	10	0	7	36	6	15	0	0	1	0.525	0.034	0.077	0.284	0.023	0.057	5.57	5
		exp.	2[illegible]7.1	35.4	82.6	5.3	1.2	6.6	36.1	5.9	14.5	0.2	1.2	1.5								
Dama[12]	119	obs.	[illegible]0	9	21	0	0	3	3	0	3	0	0	0	0.673	0.035	0.071	0.152	0.000	0.069	3.93	5
		exp.	[illegible].2	6.9	25.0	1.2	0.1	1.8	2.7	0	2.5	0	0	0.6								
Kwengo[14]	35	obs.	[illegible]	5	4	0	0	2	0	0	0	0	0	0	0.828	0.082	0.090	0.000	0.000	0.000	1.29	1
		exp.	[illegible].0	4.8	5.2	0.5	0.2	0.3	0	0	0	0	0	0								
Denasena[15]	77	obs.	[illegible]	4	8	0	0	4	3	0	0	0	0	0	0.689	0.029	0.093	0.189	0.000	0.000	0.94[a]	1
		exp.	5[illegible].1	4.0	12.8	0.4	0.1	0.7	2.8	0	0	0	0	0								

[a] Derived by pooling apparent homozygotes for R^2 with heterozygotes (see text).

Table XIc. The V factor of the rhesus system

Population	n	Phenotypes					Gene frequency:
		V(–)	V(+)				*V*
			ccDee	CcDee	ccDEe	ccdee	
San							
G/wi	36	28	7	1	0	0	0.111
G//ana	31	23	7	0	1	0	0.139
Nharo	147	96	47	1	2	1	0.188
//au//en	210	149	58	2	1	0	0.158
!Kung, Dobe	383	259	103	12	0	9	0.178
!Kung, /ai/ai	63	43	16	2	0	2	0.174
Khoi							
Topnaar, Sesfontein	42	40	2	0	0	0	0.024
Negro							
Dama	52	43	9	0	0	0	0.091

would be as follows: $r = 0.189$, $R^0 = 0.514$, $R^1 = 0.027$, $R^2 = 0.078$, $cD\text{-} = 0.192$, $\chi^2_{[1]} = 1.0$.

Other clinical conditions associated with the rhesus system involve auto-haemolysis and are associated either with a defect of antigen on the red cell surface or with the administration of drugs. The hunter-gatherers of Southern Africa are unlikely to be exposed very soon to the sophisticated perils of methyl-dopa, not only on account of their remoteness but also because of the apparent absence or extreme rarity of hypertension among them (chapter 5). The poor χ^2 fit with Hardy-Weinberg equilibrium shown for this system by two neighbouring San populations, the Northern and Ngami !Kung, could be accounted for by postulating a low-frequency *–De* or *–D–* allele, though inbreeding not disclosed by questioning of subjects seems a more probably explanation. It would not appear that either of the alleles suggested is associated with haemolysis even when homozygous, though in a parous woman such homozygosity would of course add to the danger of producing a child with haemolytic disease of the newborn.

117 San have been tested by JENKINS [1972] for the C^w antigen without a single positive being found. No other Southern African hunter-gatherers have been investigated for this antigen. JENKINS [1972] also established by family studies that the V(ce^s) antigen is associated in the San with the *r* allele as well as with *cDe*. From the frequencies shown in table XIc it will be seen that the distribution in all the hunter-gatherer peoples tested is consistent with these findings.

The P Blood Group and Helminthiasis

The presence of P_1-like substance in some parasitic worms, and the possibility that $P_1(-)$ individuals would consequently be better able to form antibodies against them, are discussed by RACE and SANGER [1968]. HEINZ [1962] demonstrated small numbers of hookworms in Central Kalahari San, and METZ *et al.* [1971] showed infestation of 3 out of 18 !Kung with *Necator americanus.* No other intestinal helminths have been reported. The only San populations investigated for P_1 are the !Xõ, with 1 negative out of 51 and thus a P^1 gene frequency of 0.860, the 36 ǂhuã:, among whom all were positive, and 277 Tsumkwe !Kung, where the 36 negatives produced a P^1 frequency of 0.639. Of the 92 Dama tested, 4 were negative, giving a gene frequency for P^1 of 0.792. There are no data about helminthiasis in the Kuiseb Topnaar, whose P^1 frequency is the low one of 0.491, derived from 15 negatives of 58 tested. It is perhaps significant that they do keep goats; it would be interesting to know whether hydatid disease occurs.

The ABH Secretor Status and the Lewis Blood Groups

An association has been demonstrated between the inability to secrete ABH substance in the saliva and the occurrence of duodenal ulcer (MCCONNELL, 1966]. The secretor polymorphism is included here because of its association with the Lewis blood groups and because, like the other polymorphisms in this section, it is detected by an immunological technique. Nothing is known about peptic ulceration in any of the hunter-gatherer populations of Southern Africa, and no evidence of its presence among the !Kung was collected by BRONTË-STEWART *et al.* [1960] or TRUSWELL and HANSEN [1975]; there is, however, a fair amount of data about the ABH secretor status of some of these, beginning with the study by JENKINS and CLEATON-JONES [1966], and these data and what is known of the Lewis phenotypes and gene frequencies are shown in table XII. It will be seen that the phenotype Le(a+b+), not usually found in adults but reported among Australian aborigines (MOURANT, personal commun.], does occur in the San, and that some Le(a+) individuals appear to be secretors and some Le(a−b+) individuals to be non-secretors. It is possible that apparent secretion could be due to the chewing of vegetable matter containing ABH-like substances shortly before the saliva was collected; it is less easy to explain the last-mentioned exceptions.

There is a great variation of frequencies of *Le* and *Se* among these groups, but nothing much can be made of them anthropologically or medically in the absence of other data.

Table XII. Secretor and Lewis phenotypes and gene frequencies

Population	n	Phenotypes														Gene frequencies			
		Le(a+b–)			Le(a+b+)			Le(a–b+)			Le(a–b–)			Lewis not known		secretor		Lewis	
		S	N	U	S	N	U	S	N	U	S	N	U	S	N	*Se*	*se*	*Le*	*le*
San																			
Central + Southern[6]	86	–	–	–	–	–	–	–	–	–	–	–	–	84	2	0.848	0.152	–	–
Southern, mainly !Xõ[6]	60	1	5	0	0	0	–	46	0	–	8	0	–	–	–	0.724	0.276	0.635	0.365
Nharo[6]	106	3	1	8	1	0	1	22	0	47	14	2	17	–	–	0.916	0.084	0.530	0.470
//au//en[6]	94	2	1	1	0	0	0	9	0	1	3	0	1	53	23	0.514	0.486	0.553	0.447
!Kung, Ngami[6]	152	–	–	–	–	–	–	–	–	–	–	–	–	142	10	0.744	0.256	–	–
!Kung, Dobe[6]	350	7	18	6	5	1	1	87	6	25	50	9	10	105	20	0.582	0.418	0.437	0.563
!Kung, /ai/ai[6]	65	0	5	1	0	0	0	27	0	0	16	2	4	–	–	0.658	0.342	0.419	0.581
!Kung, /du/da[6]	87	1	2	–	0	0	–	35	0	–	2	1	–	48	7	0.661	0.339	0.646	0.354
!Kung, G!ãg!ai[6]	35	0	0	–	0	0	–	7	0	–	5	0	–	23	0	1.000	0.000	0.354	0.646
Khoi																			
Topnaar, Kuiseb[9]	58	1	[illegible]	–	–	–	–	26	0	–	3	0	–	20	0	0.611	0.389	0.679	0.321
Topnaar, Sesfontein[6]	42	0	7	–	0	0	–	29	0	–	5	1	–	–	–	0.558	0.442	0.622	0.378
Negroes																			
Dama[12]	92	–	–	–	–	–	–	–	–	–	–	–	–	64	13	0.602	0.398	–	–
Kwengo[14]	35	0	5	1	0	0	0	15	3	4	3	4	0	–	–	0.367	0.633	0.553	0.447

S = Secretor, N = non-secretor, U = secretor status unknown.

Polymorphisms of Intracellular Proteins

A surprisingly small proportion of the numerous known variants of intracellular proteins have turned out to have any bearing on health; those that do are signalized more often by having functionally defective forms which are characterized by reduction in specific activity than by actual reductions in the amount of the protein. Few of these known defective forms ever attain polymorphic frequencies in populations; where they do, it is either known or suspected that heterozygosity for the variant and normal forms of the protein confers a selective advantage which compensates for the disadvantage to the population of the occasional homozygote for the variant, and that the polymorphism is consequently a balanced one.

Many of these protein polymorphisms were first reported on in these populations by JENKINS *et al.* [1971]; the data have been incorporated, and supplemented, in JENKINS [1972].

Haemoglobins

The classical example of a balanced polymorphism is, of course, that of haemoglobin S, sickle cell haemoglobin, in parts of Africa and Asia, where heterozygosity protects against malaria. Haemoglobin C appears to confer similar protection, as do the thalassaemia polymorphisms of the Mediterranean and Asia. No hunter-gatherer populations of Southern Africa have so far produced a single instance of the presence of haemoglobins S or C, but it is to be regretted that no data are on hand concerning the Kwisi, who, if they are closely related to or intermixed with the Kuvale, might be expected to have S. The three Negro hunter-gatherer peoples in South West Africa, the Dama, Kwengo and Cimba, and the Denasena in Botswana, lack it entirely.

Another β-chain variant has been found to occur in the San, and to reach polymorphic frequencies in the //au//en, where 16 persons out of 267 had it. It is haemoglobin D Bushman [WADE *et al.*, 1966]. The gene frequency for *Hb*$\beta^{\mathrm{DBushman}}$ in the //au//en is 0.029. One of 147 Nharo, 1 of 422 Dobe !Kung and 2 of 64 !Kung from /ai/ai also possessed this variant, with gene frequencies of 0.004, 0.001 and 0.008, respectively. Haematological examinations carried out on bearers of this variant have not shown that it confers any disadvantage [JENKINS, 1972]. The equally inoffensive δ-chain variant known as haemoglobin A_2' or B_2 is known to be fairly common in the Negro Herero pastoralists of South West Africa [JENKINS, 1972], and in a very small sample of 19 probably very closely interrelated Cimba there were 8 heterozygotes and 1 homozygote [JENKINS, unpublished]. An apparent α-chain variant of very high frequency has been found among the ǂhuã: and !Xõ, in 17 out of 36 of the former and 21 out of 51 of the latter. The variant has not yet been characterized, but the possibility that it may represent a chain prolongation variant of the Hb Constant Spring type is being explored. It does not appear to be associated with any haematological disability. No thalassaemia-like conditions, or hereditary persistence of haemoglobin F, have been found in any of the Southern African hunter-gatherer peoples.

The Glucose-6-Phosphate Dehydrogenase (G6PD) Polymorphism

The intracellular enzyme G6PD catalyzes the conversion of glucose-6-phosphate to 6-phosphogluconate, a reaction which produces the NADPH necessary for the maintenance of glutathione in a reduced state and hence for the preservation of red cell integrity. Where the naturally occurring enzyme is deficient in activity, any induced reduction of the activity can lead to haemolysis. Deficiency is found at polymorphic frequencies in a number of populations which are or have been exposed to malaria, and is held to protect against that condition by causing the cells containing the parasite to haemolyze before intraerythrocytic maturation is complete. The characteristically African forms of the enzyme consist of the usual B, the African deficient isoenzyme A^-, and the A variant which has almost as much activity as B but is claimed also to give some protection against malaria [BIENZLE *et al.*, 1972]. A number of oxidizing drugs, including some administered for malaria, also can provoke haemolysis where G6PD activity is deficient, and consequently need to be administered with care in populations in which deficiency occurs. The structural locus for the enzyme is on the X-chromosome, and the phenotypic frequencies in the hemizygous males consequently may be expected to be equal to the gene frequencies in the populations.

From the figures in table XIII it will be seen that the finding by CHARLTON and BOTHWELL [1961] that G6PD deficiency was much less common in San than in Negro populations has been abundantly confirmed. Both of the characteristically Negro variants, however, are found; this is probably due to admixture. Many Southern African populations, particularly Negro and Coloured (Mixed) ones, display a curious anomaly in the distribution of the variants; there is an excess of A homozygotes among females which cannot be accounted for by random inactivation of the X-chromosome [NURSE and JENKINS, 1973b]. The anomaly is shown by only two of the non-Negro hunter-gatherer peoples, the related G/wi and G//ana, who show other evidences of Negro admixture [JENKINS *et al.*, 1975]. Among the Negroes, it

Table XIII. G6PD phenotypes and gene frequencies

Population		Phenotypes										Gene frequencies[a]				χ^2[1]
		males					females									
		n	A	A⁻	B	Bwk	n	AA+ AA⁻	A⁻A⁻	AB+ A⁻B	BB	*Gd*A	*Gd*A⁻	*Gd*B	*Gd*Bwk	
San																
G!aokx'ate[10]	obs.	18	0	0	18	0	15	0	0	0	15	0.000	0.000	1.000	0.000	–
	exp.		–	–	–	–	–	–	–	–	–					
!Xõ[16]	obs.	28	0	0	27	1	23	0	0	0	23	0.000	0.000	0.964	0.036	–
	exp.		0	0	27.0	1.0		0	0	0	23.0					
ǂhuã[13]	obs.	12	1	1	9	1	23	0	0	1	22	0.026	0.026	0.876	0.072	8.92
	exp.		0.3	0.3	10.5	0.9		0.0	0.0	2.3	20.7					
G/wi[7]	obs.	47	0	1	46	0	47	1	0	0	46	0.009	0.012	0.979	0.000	very large
	exp.		0.4	0.6	46.0	0		0.01	0.0	1.9	45.1					
G//ana[7]	obs.	25	1	0	24	0	25	1	0	0	24	0.040	0.000	0.960	0.000	very large
	exp.		1.0	0	24.0	0		0.04	0	1.9	23.1					
Nharo[6]	obs.	19	2	1	16	0	21	0	0	0	21	0.033	0.016	0.951	0.000	7.23
	exp.		0.6	0.3	18.1	0		0.0	0.0	2.0	19.0					
//au//en[6]	obs.	32	0	0	32	0	28	0	0	1	27	0.011	0.000	0.989	0.000	1.32
	exp.		0.4	0	31.6	0		0.0	0	0.6	27.4					
!Kung, Dobe[6]	obs.	94	4	1	89	0	110	0	0	10	100	0.038	0.010	0.952	0.000	0.20
	exp.		3.6	0.9	89.5	0		0.2	0.0	10.1	99.7					
!Kung, /du/da[6]	obs.	27	0	1	26	0	20	0	0	0	20	0.000	0.037	0.963	0.000	1.53
	exp.		0	1.0	26.0	0		0	0.0	1.4	18.5					
!Kung, Tsumkwe[6]	obs.	69	5	0	64	0	77	2	0	2	73	0.049	0.000	0.951	0.000	20.91
	exp.		3.4	0	65.6	0		0.2	0	7.2	69.6					
!Kung, G!ãg!ai[10]	obs.	14	1	0	13	0	22	0	0	1	21	0.034	0.000	0.966	0.000	0.70
	exp.		0.5	0	13.5	0		0.0	0	1.4	20.5					
Khoi																
Topnaar, Kuiseb[9]	obs.	25	0	0	25	0	23	0	0	3	20	0.042	0.000	0.958	0.000	1.84
	exp.		1.1	0	23.9	0		0.0	0	1.9	21.1					
Topnaar, Sesfontein[6]	obs.	20	0	0	20	0	22	0	0	0	22	0.000	0.000	1.000	0.000	–
	exp.		–	–	–	–		–	–	–	–					
Negro																
Dama[12]	obs.	63	11	1	51	0	56	0	0	12	44	0.126	0.011	0.863	0.000	2.90
	exp.		7.9	0.7	54.4	0		1.0	0.0	13.2	41.7					
Kwengo[14]	obs.	20	7	1	12	0	15	3	0	3	9	0.301	0.039	0.660	0.000	4.32
	exp.		6.0	0.8	13.2	0		1.7	0.0	6.7	6.5					
Denasena[15]	obs.	36	2	0	34	0	41	4	0	6	31	0.136	0.000	0.864	0.000	16.14
	exp.		4.9	0	31.1	0		0.8	0	9.6	30.6					

[a] Calculated by a modification of the method of HALDANE [1963].

is present in the Kwengo, in whom small sample size might be responsible, and in the Denasena, where the sample size was adequate. The three other San populations for which a significant χ^2 value is found show a deficiency of female A and AB phenotypes. This question is currently being investigated.

Adenosine Deaminase and Immune Deficiency

It has been found that some cases of severe combined immunological deficiency are associated with low levels or absence of erythrocyte adenosine deaminase [GIBLETT *et al.,* 1972). Apparent absence of this enzyme from the red cells has been reported in one healthy !Kung boy from Tsumkwe [JENKINS, 1973]. Subsequent studies have shown that both his parents have reduced red cell adenosine deaminase activity, and that a similar reduction of activity is found also in a number of random unrelated members of the same population. The allele determining the deficiency, ADA^8, appears to be present at polymorphic frequencies, 0.154 ± 0.027 [JENKINS *et al.,* publication pending]. Corroborative evidence for this has been provided lately by the finding of an unrelated boy with the same condition. Small amounts of the enzyme are present in the red cells of affected individuals; white cell lysates and cultured fibroblasts show a weak ADA1 pattern on electrophoresis. The proband shows no sign of severe immunological defect [JENKINS *et al.,* publication pending]. The variant has not yet been detected in any other San or Khoi population, or in Negro hunter-gatherers.

The common variant ADA^2 does not reach polymorphic frequencies in most Southern African populations so far tested. It appears to be absent from most; consequently, no table has been compiled for this system. Besides the Tsumkwe population, the !Xõ, ǂhuã:, G/wi, G//ana, G!ãg!ai, G!aokx'ate, Hei//om, Dama, Kwengo and Denasena among hunter-gatherers have been tested for it. Apart from a single ADA2–1 individual in the large Tsumkwe sample, two unidentified electrophoretic variants among the G!ãg!ai, and two individuals who gave weakly staining patterns among the ǂhuã:, the only variant detected was the weak one described above.

Serum Protein Polymorphisms

Four clinically relevant serum protein polymorphisms have been investigated in Southern African hunter-gatherer populations. The pseudocholinesterase variation determined at the E_1 locus is important in anaesthesia; it has been investigated in one San population, a small mixed sample consisting mainly of !Xõ, one Khoi hunter-gatherer population, the Topnaar of the Kuiseb Valley, and the Dama, without any variant form of the enzyme being found [JENKINS, 1972]. The other three systems show more variation.

Haptoglobins

The haptoglobins are α_2-globulins possessing the property of binding haemoglobin; the resultant complex is removed from the circulation by the reticulo-endothelial system. The circulating haptoglobin consequently tends to become depleted in haemolytic states, and its quantitative estimation can be of diagnostic value. It is also well established that there is a seasonal fluctuation in haptoglobin levels in some populations, and that this appears to be related either to food intake or to malaria or both. Anhaptoglobinaemia is found in high phenotypic frequencies in Negroes, and it has been suggested that it has a negative population association with the 2–1 mod. phenotype also common in them. There is a rare genetic amorph, the presence of which in Africa has never been established; a possible reason for the high frequency of Hp^1 in Negroes may be a selective operation of environmental factors on phenotypes determined by the Hp^2 allele and thus possessing lower absolute

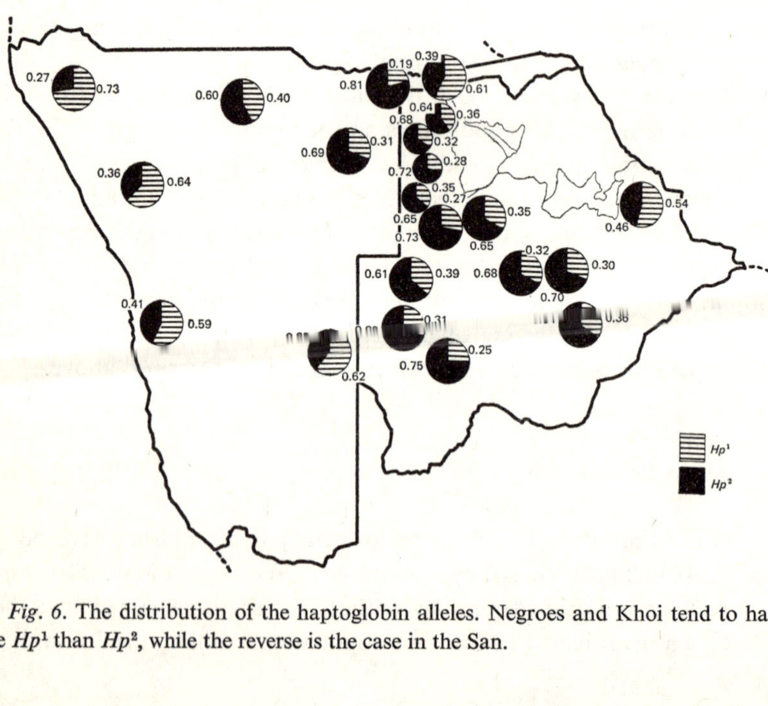

Fig. 6. The distribution of the haptoglobin alleles. Negroes and Khoi tend to have more Hp^1 than Hp^2, while the reverse is the case in the San.

quantities of the protein, so that the apparent anhaptoglobinaemics are in fact genotypically Hp^2/Hp^2 or Hp^1/Hp^2. A survey of changes in seasonal haptoglobin patterns in a small sample of !Kung provides some support for this [JENKINS, 1972].

A search for possible haptoglobin-ABO blood group interaction in 156 San families failed to disclose the excess of Hpl phenotypes in the children of ABO incompatible matings reported in other populations. It was, however, observed that there was a significantly higher frequency of surviving HpO children born to ABO compatible than to ABO incompatible matings [JENKINS, 1972], which might be accounted for by a relatively greater mortality among neonates with genetically lower haptoglobin levels. A recent study by VANA and STEINBERG [1975] has, nonetheless, furnished evidence that ABO incompatibility plays no part in the interaction. They found that in two North American Caucasoid isolates there were significantly higher frequencies of Hp^1 among individuals not of group O, and that the frequencies appeared to be inversely related to the number of O alleles in the genotype. By far the largest number of ABO compatible matings in any population are OxO, and the higher Hp^1 frequency among ABO incompatible matings could be accounted for by a negative association of Hp^1 with group O. The association may, they admit, not exist in all populations; but it certainly could be invoked to account for any ostensible connection between haptoglobin type and the offspring of particular mating classes.

It can be seen from tables XIVa and b that Hp^1 frequencies are very much higher in Negro and Khoi hunter-gatherer populations than in the San, and this is irrespective of the proportion of HpO phenotypes. The haptoglobin frequencies in the Hei//om are in the San rather than the Khoi range, and suggest that the category in which we have considered them here may in fact be erroneous. On the other hand, the Denasena frequencies are barely Khoi or Negro, but the weight of all the other evidence that the Denasena are Negro tends to make us discount the suggestion of considerable San admixture provided in this single system. The lowest frequency Hp^1 found was in the G!ãg!ai !Kung, admittedly a very small sample but one which also contained the highest proportion (0.25) of HpO individuals. An interesting trend which does emerge from tables XIVa and b is the purely geographical one of higher HpO frequencies in the northernmost samples irrespective of race; though it must be pointed out that the Khoi of Sesfontein and the Hei//om are exceptions to this. Malaria is certainly more prevalent in the northern populations, excluding that at Sesfontein. Furthermore, the χ^2 agreement with Hardy-Weinberg expectations is good for all,

Table XIVa. Haptoglobin phenotypes and gene frequencies in the San

Population	n		Phenotypes					Gene frequencies		$\chi^2_{[1]}$
			1	2–1	2–1 mod.	2	0	*Hp*[1]	*Hp*[2]	
G!aokx'ate[10]	33	obs.	11	19	0	3	0	0.621	0.379	1.58
		exp.	12.7	15.6		4.7				
Southern, mainly !Xõ[6]	70	obs.	7	22	3	37	1	0.311	0.689	0.24
		exp.	5.8	28.4		34.8				
!Xõ[16]	50	obs.	2	21	0	27	0	0.250	0.750	0.69
		exp.	3.1	18.8		28.1				
ǂhuã:[13]	33	obs.	5	14	0	14	0	0.364	0.636	0.25
		exp.	4.4	15.3		13.3				
G/wi[1]	94	obs.	10	36	2	44	2	0.315	0.685	0.18
		exp.	9.1	39.7		43.2				
G//ana[7]	50	obs.	3	23	0	22	2	0.302	0.698	0.92
		exp.	4.4	20.2		23.4				
Nharo[6]	147	obs.	23	65	3	56	0	0.388	0.612	0.10
		exp.	22.1	69.8		55.1				
//au//en[6]	265	obs.	19	101	2	137	6	0.272	0.728	0.00
		exp.	19.2	102.6		137.2				
!Kung, northern[6]	85	obs.	9	36	1	31	8	0.357	0.643	0.16
		exp.	9.8	35.4		31.8				
!Kung, Ngami[6]	173	obs.	20	69	2	60	22	0.347	0.653	2.62
		exp.	15.8	59.4		55.8				
!Kung, Dobe[6]	423	obs.	38	155	5	173	52	0.318	0.682	0.01
		exp.	37.5	160.9		172.5				
!Kung, /ai/ai[6]	60	obs.	8	20	0	24	8	0.346	0.654	1.12
		exp.	6.2	23.5		22.2				
!Kung, /du/da[6]	101	obs.	5	43	0	48	5	0.276	0.724	1.38
		exp.	7.3	38.4		50.3				
!Kung, Tsumkwe[6]	272	obs.	21	111	4	118	18	0.309	0.691	0.60
		exp.	24.2	108.5		121.3				
!Kung, G!ãg!ai[10]	36	obs.	0	7	3	17	9	0.185	0.815	1.40
		exp.	0.9	8.1		17.9				

Gene frequencies, expected numbers and χ^2 calculated by pooling the 2–1 and 2–1 mod. phenotypes excluding HpO.

and exceptionally good for most, populations. It would not seem that the gene frequency differences are appreciably related to preferential depletion of haptoglobin in Hp2 individuals, but rather that they do represent an actual racial difference, except perhaps in the cases of the Denasena and the Hei//om, where the operation of drift might be invoked.

Transferrins

The transferrins are β-globulins which take up from the reticuloendothelial cells the iron from catabolized haemoglobin and transport it to the

Table XIVb. Haptoglobin phenotypes and gene frequencies in the Khoi and Negroes

Population	n		Phenotypes					Gene frequencies		$\chi^2_{[1]}$
			1	2–1	2–1 mod.	2	0	*Hp*[1]	*Hp*[2]	
Khoi										
Topnaar, Kuiseb[9]	58	obs.	17	34	0	7	0	0.586	0.414	2.47
		exp.	19.9	28.8		9.9				
Topnaar, Sesfontein[6]	42	obs.	20	20	1	1	0	0.726	0.274	2.84
		exp.	22.2	16.7		3.2				
Hei//om[10]	87	obs.	16	47	0	24	0	0.397	0.603	2.89
		exp.	13.7	41.7	0	31.6				
Negro										
Dama[12]	117	obs.	49	36	9	17	6	0.644	0.356	1.48
		exp.	46.0	50.9		14.1				
Kwengo[14]	35	obs.	10	11	3	4	7	0.607	0.393	0.06
		exp.	10.3	13.4	4.3					
Denasena[15]	79	obs.	17	26	7	12	17	0.540	0.460	0.32
		exp.	18.1	30.8		13.1				

Gene frequencies, expected numbers and χ^2 calculated by pooling the Hp 2–1 and Hp 2–1 mod. phenotypes and excluding HpO.

bone marrow for reincorporation into haemoglobin. They are also concerned with the transport of dietary iron after intestinal absorption; they are required for the selective delivery of iron to red cell precursors [Bothwell and Finch, 1962]. It has been suggested that they exert a bacteriostatic effect by competing for iron with certain bacteria [Rogers, 1967].

As can be seen from table XV, the transferrin D_1 variant attains high frequencies among the northern San while in the other populations it either is not found or the frequencies are appreciably lower. It has been established [Kirk *et al.*, 1964; Wang *et al.*, 1967] that the Negro D_1 variant is electrophoretically and chemically identical with that found among Australasian hunter-gatherers. In Southern Africa, it seems to represent an essentially San character, and its presence in other peoples can be ascribed to San admixture. That identical mutations should ostensibly have taken place in desert-dwelling populations so remote from one another and apparently with no very recent common origin strongly suggests that the variant must present a selective advantage in desert environments, but it is not yet clear what this advantage is. It has been shown that the total iron-binding capacity of the transferrin CD_1 heterozygote is significantly lower than that of the normal C homozygote [Jenkins, 1972], but further work is needed to establish the relevance of this.

Table XV. Transferrin phenotypes and gene frequencies

Population	n		Phenotypes			Gene frequencies		χ^2[1]
			CC	CD_1	D_1D_1	Tf^C	Tf^{D_1}	
San								
G!aokx'ate[10]	33		33	0	0	1.000	0.000	
Southern, mainly !Xõ[6]	70		60	10	0	0.929	0.071	0.47
!Xõ[16]	50		44	6	0	0.940	0.060	0.23
ǂhuã:[13]	35		35	0	0	1.000	0.000	
G/wi[7]	93		87	6	0	0.968	0.032	0.11
G//ana[7]	50		49	1	0	0.990	0.010	0.00
Nharo[6]	147	obs.	124	22	1	0.918	0.082	0.00
		exp.	124.0	22.0	1.0			
//au//en[6]	265	obs.	220	44	1	0.913	0.087	0.60
		exp.	221.0	42.0	2.0			
!Kung, northern[6]	87	obs.	58	27	2	0.822	0.178	0.28
		exp.	58.8	25.5	2.7			
!Kung, Ngami[6]	153	obs.	122	30	1	0.895	0.105	0.35
		exp.	122.7	28.7	1.7			
!Kung, Dobe[6]	418	obs.	301	107	10	0.848	0.152	0.01
		exp.	300.7	107.7	9.7			
!Kung, /ai/ai[6]	60	obs.	36	22	2	0.783	0.217	0.37
		exp.	36.8	20.4	2.8			
!Kung, /du/da[6]	101	obs.	57	38	6	0.752	0.248	0.01
		exp.	57.2	37.6	6.2			
!Kung, Tsumkwe[6]	272	obs.	192	70	10	0.834	0.166	1.25
		exp.	189.2	75.3	7.5			
!Kung, G!ãg!ai[10]	36		31	5	0	0.931	0.069	0.20
Khoi								
Topnaar, Kuiseb[9]	58		58	0	0	1.000	0.000	
Topnaar, Sesfontein[6]	42		41	1	0	0.988	0.012	0.00
Negro								
Dama[12]	117		117	0	0	1.000	0.000	
Kwengo[14]	35		34	1	0	0.986	0.014	0.06
Denasena[15]	79		75	4	0	0.949	0.051	

The 'Group-Specific Component' or Gc

Another α_2-globulin besides haptoglobin has been shown to be polymorphic in most populations; it is called Gc. Very few data exist for Southern African populations and nothing is known about its possible function in the body apart from an unconfirmed finding that Gc combines with vitamin D [CAVALLI-SFORZA, 1974, personal commun. to MOURANT]. A small number (72) of Southern San (mainly !Xõ) have been tested for Gc and 54 were found to be Gcl, 18 were Gc2–1 and there were no Gc2 individuals, giving a Gc^2 allele frequency of 0.125 [JENKINS and BARNICOT, 1968]. This frequency is very little different from that found in Zulu by MCDERMID and VOS [1971] and in Zambians by KITCHIN and BEARN [1966]. The Gc^{Ab} allele, which gives a faster moving Gc pattern than the Gc^{1} allele, was not found in the San, although it attained frequencies of 0.036 in the Zulu and 0.03 in the Lenje of Zambia.

Chapter 4. Polymorphisms of No Known Medical Relevance

The search for information of anthropological interest has in the past been the main incentive for the investigation of genetic polymorphisms which appeared to lack any clinical significance. A number of the blood groups are of very little interest or importance from the standpoint of blood transfusion or of association with disease, and comparatively few of the erythrocyte enzyme systems have been shown to maintain at polymorphic frequencies variants with a known bearing on health. The field of the serum proteins has not been extensively explored as yet in Southern African hunter-gatherer populations, and it is particularly regrettable that so little is known about such medically significant systems as complement, α_1-antitrypsin and ceruloplasmin in these peoples. On the other hand, the immunoglobulins have been investigated and shown to be of great anthropological importance.

Red Cell Antigen Systems

MNSs and Henshaw

A number of polymorphic red cell antigens are known to be associated in close linkage with the MNSs system. The choice of which are to be investigated naturally depends on the availability of the particular sera; one, the Henshaw antigen, has proved very suitable for study in Southern Africa. The allele determining this antigen is found in coupling with various of the MNSs alleles in various African populations. In West Africa, the linkage appears to be primarily with *NS* [Chalmers *et al.*, 1953], whereas in Zaire it is with *MS* [Nijenhuis, 1953]. In 1953, again, Zoutendyk *et al.* showed coupling with *NS* in the San and in 1955 that in the Khoi it was linked to *MS*. Subsequent studies, the particulars of which are shown in tables XVIa and b, have shown coupling in the various San populations with *MS, NS* and *Ns,* but not with *Ms*. Coupling with *Ns* is uncommon; it is phenotypically obvious in only two populations, the Dobe !Kung and the Hei//om, but appears on maximum likelihood estimations probably to be present also

Table XVIa. The MNS and Henshaw blood group phenotypes and gene frequencies in the San

Population	n		Phenotypes: MMS	MMSHe	MMss	MNS	MNSHe	MNss	MNssHe	NNS	NNSHe	NNss	NNssHe	Gene frequencies: *MS*	*MSHe*	*Ms*	*NS*	*NSHe*	*Ns*	*NsHe*	χ^{2a}	d.f.
G!aokx'ate[10]	33	obs.	1	8	2	5	3	12	0	1	0	1	0	0.056	0.149	0.417	0.057	0.000	0.321	0.000	10.32	5
		exp.	1.6	5.4	5.7	3.0	3.8	8.8	0	1.3	0	3.4	0									
!Xõ[16]	51	obs.	2	4	14	1	1	23	0	0	0	6	0	0.033	0.049	0.555	0.000	0.000	0.363	0.000	1.18	3
		exp.	1.9	3.1	15.7	1.2	1.8	20.5	0	0	0	6.7	0									
ǂhuã[13]	36	obs.	2	1	8	2	0	11	0	1	1	9	0	0.046	0.014	0.426	0.058	0.014	0.442	0.000	4.56	3
		exp.	1.5	0.5	6.5	3.4	0.9	13.6	0	2.0	0.5	7.0	0									
G/wi[7]	94	obs.	6	2	21	12	2	32	0	3	0	16	0	0.068	0.022	0.489	0.048	0.000	0.373	0.000	2.06	3
		exp.	6.8	2.3	22.5	9.8	1.7	34.3	0	3.6	0	13.1	0									
G//ana[7]	50	obs.	10	0	13	10	3	9	0	2	0	3	0	0.164	0.028	0.507	0.037	0.000	0.264	0.000	4.07[b]	2
		exp.	9.7	1.9	12.9	6.8	0.8	13.4	0	1.0	0	3.5	0									
Nharo[6]	125	obs.	10	10	32	14	2	45	0	0	0	12	0	0.095	0.060	0.505	0.000	0.000	0.340	0.000	7.48	3
		exp.	13.0	9.4	31.9	8.1	5.1	42.9	0	0	0	14.5	0									
//au//en[6]	111	obs.	3	10	17	7	11	32	1	2	6	22	0	0.042	0.081	0.377	0.024	0.000	0.431	0.045	3.90[c]	4
		exp.	3.7	8.3	15.8	6.2	9.5	36.1	3.8	2.4	0.2	20.6	4.5									
!Kung, northern[6]	103	obs.	13		19	11		40		3		17		0.113		0.446	0.029		0.413		0.76	2
		exp.	11.7		20.5	12.9		37.9		2.5		17.6										
!Kung, Ngami[6]	58	obs.	3		8	5		32		0		10		0.071		0.438	0.000		0.491		4.44	2
		exp.	3.9		11.1	4.0		24.9		0		14.0										
!Kung, Dobe[6]	258	obs.	7	[illegible]8	58	13	29	75	0	4	2	52	2	0.028	0.093	0.432	0.027	0.000	0.409	0.011	11.75	3
		exp.	6.4	24.3	48.1	12.3	21.6	91.2	2.5	5.9	0.2	43.2	2.3									
!Kung, /ai/ai[6]	65	obs.	2	3	17	2	2	27	0	0	1	11	0	0.025	0.040	0.512	0.000	0.016	0.407	0.000	0.96	3
		exp.	1.7	2.9	17.0	1.3	3.3	27.1	0	0	0.9	10.8	0									
!Kung, /du/da[6]	64	obs.	1	1	6	4	2	24	0	2	0	24	0	0.020	0.019	0.305	0.018	0.000	0.638	0.000	1.45	3
		exp.	0.8	0.8	6.0	2.4	1.6	24.9	0	1.5	0	26.1	0									
!Kung, Tsumkwe[6]	248	obs.	3	4	44	8	13	109	0	1	4	62	0	0.021	0.023	0.424	0.012	0.013	0.508	0.000	4.31	3
		exp.	4.5	5.2	44.6	7.8	8.9	106.8	0	3.0	3.3	64.0	0									
!Kung, G!ãg!ai[10]	36	obs.	1	0	5	0	3	12	0	0	0	15	0	0.027	0.024	0.320	0.000	0.000	0.629	0.000	5.04	3
		exp.	0.6	0.6	3.7	12	1.1	14.5	0	0	0	14.2	0									

[a] Derived by pooling categories in which the expected value is less than 1.

[b] Derived by pooling He(+) phenotypes.

[c] Derived by pooling expected phenotypes for which *NsHe* would inequivocally be responsible.

Table XVIb. MNS and Henshaw blood group phenotypes and gene frequencies in Khoi and Negroes

Population	n		Phenotypes											Gene frequencies							χ^2	d.f.
			MMS	MMSHe	MMss	MNS	MNSHe	MNss	MNssHe	NNS	NNSHe	NNss	NNssHe	*MS*	*MSHe*	*Ms*	*NS*	*NSHe*	*Ns*	*NsHe*		
Khoi																						
Topnaar, Kuiseb[9]	58[14]	obs.	(3)	25	(1)	(4)	30		(6)	(0)	3		(0)		0.690				0.310		2.54	1
		exp.		27.6			24.8				5.6											
Topnaar, Sesfontein[6]	42	obs.	1	2	3	4	4	15	0	2	3	8	0	0.071	0.059	0.345	0.048	0.000	0.441	0.036	6.58[a]	4
		exp.	2.3	2.2	5.0	4.3	2.8	12.8	1.0	1.9	0.1	8.2	1.4									
Hei//om[10]	96	obs.	9	5	19	7	7	37	0	0	0	11	1	0.119	0.065	0.440	0.000	0.000	0.347	0.029	4.03	3
		exp.	11.4	7.4	18.6	7.9	5.4	29.3	2.4	0	0	11.6	2.0									
Negro																						
Dama[11]	448	obs.		91			221					136			0.450				0.550		0.00	1
		exp.		90.7			221.8					135.5										
Dama[12]	119	obs.	5	0	17	9	1	51	0	5	4	27	0	0.046	0.000	0.394	0.063	0.025	0.472	0.000	3.93	3
		exp.	4.6	0	18.5	11.7	2.6	44.3	0	7.5	3.3	26.5	0									
Kwengo[14]	35	obs.	6	1	14	3	1	8	0	0	0	2	0	0.141	0.029	0.592	0.000	0.000	0.238	0.000	1.52	3
		exp.	6.5	1.5	12.3	2.3	0.5	9.9	0	0	0	2.0	0									
Denasena[15]	77	obs.	1	0	24	3	0	33	0	3	0	15	0	0.019	0.000	0.525	0.032	0.000	0.424	0.000	5.14	3
		exp.	1.6	0	21.8	4.8	0	35.2	0	2.2	0	14.2	0									

[a] Derived by pooling expected values for which *NsHe* would be responsible.

in the Sesfontein Khoi and the //au//en. In the light of ZOUTENDYK *et al.*'s finding, it is somewhat surprising that such low frequencies of *NSHe* should be calculated for the San populations in which it is known to occur, while San frequencies of *MSHe* are comparatively high. The expected coupling with *MS* is also evident in the Khoi and Kwengo, but in the Dama the coupling is unequivocally with *NS*. The Denasena appear not to possess the antigen at all; it was found neither in the 77 members of the random sample nor in 43 of their kinsfolk.

Frequencies of *NS* are low in all of these populations, and from some it is absent. If it is genuinely absent from the Kwengo, a Negro population, as well as from several Khoisan ones, it could be suggested that such low frequencies must be due to unidentified selective factors rather than to drift; but the Kwengo sample, consisting entirely of unrelated individuals, is very small. If such selective factors exist, they would seem to operate least on the G!aokx'ate, Dama, ǂhuã:, G/wi, G//ana and the Sesfontein Khoi, who share no common environmental factor not equally applicable to the other populations.

In some populations, better agreement with Hardy-Weinberg expectations is obtained when the results of testing with anti-s are disregarded. This may be due to the notorious unreliability of such sera or to the presence of an allele determining N but neither S nor s, the so-called NS^{u} allele. Such an allele could in its homozygous state be detected by the failure of the red cells to agglutinate in the presence of an anti-u serum, which detects a factor common to S and s. The !Xõ, ǂhuã:, G/wi, G//ana, G!ãg!ai !Kung, Hei//om, Dama and Kwengo have been tested with an anti-u serum kindly supplied by Miss PHYLLIS MOORES of the Natal Blood Transfusion Service, and not a single negative case has been found. With samples of this size, however, this is hardly surprising, and it remains possible that the allele is present.

Kidd

Antisera for the Kidd antigens have not been readily available to workers in Southern Africa, and only six hunter-gatherer populations have been tested for the Jk(b) antigen. Of the 127 Nharo tested, 26 were Jk(b+), giving a gene frequency of 0.108. Among the //au//en 15 of 54 were positive, and the gene frequency was 0.150. Three !Kung populations have been tested, with 72 out of 340 positive in Dobe, 16 out of 64 in /ai/ai, and 6 out of 47 in /du/da. The respective gene frequencies are 0.112, 0.134 and 0.066. There were 94 Hei//om tested, with only 17 positive, and a gene frequency of 0.093.

Table XVII. Xg phenotypes and gene frequencies

Population	n		Xg phenotypes				Gene frequencies		χ^2	d.f.
			males		females					
			Xg(a+)	Xg(a–)	Xg(a+)	Xg(a–)	*Xg*^{a}	*Xg*		
San										
!Xõ[16]	37	obs.	10	11	5	11	0.300	0.700	5.07	1
		exp.	6.3	14.7	8.2	7.8				
‡huã:[13]	32	obs.	6	4	14	8	0.444	0.556	1.35	1
		exp.	4.4	5.6	15.2	6.8				
Khoi										
Hei//om[10]	94	obs.	21	31	28	14	0.414	0.586	0.05	1
		exp.	21.5	30.5	27.6	14.4				
Negro										
Dama[12]	69	obs.	12	23	18	16	0.325	0.675	0.08	1
		exp.	11.4	23.6	18.5	15.5				

Gene frequencies calculated by the maximum likelihood method of HALDANE [1963].

In the absence of further data, these results are of little anthropological interest; it appears simply that the San have *Jk*^{b} frequencies about a quarter those of Caucasoids but within the range for Southern African Negroes [JENKINS, 1972].

Xg

The X-linked Xg blood group has only been tested for in four of these populations, shortage of antisera being once more the limiting factor. The results are shown in table XVII. The apparent significant excess of Xg(a–) females in the ‡huã: sample is probably due to incorporation of a number of closely related individuals in the sample; the reasons for this will be discussed in the section on Population Structure below.

Red Cell Enzyme Systems

These systems have turned out to be of considerable anthropological interest. They are more readily investigated than some of the red cell antigen systems for which antisera are hard to procure or for which the antisera available do not fully determine the range of genotypes. For example, to make a full investigation of the rhesus system in African populations needs an anti-V and an anti-e^S serum, neither of them easy to obtain, and without which the system appears to present comparatively little variation. Electrophoretic determination of enzyme variation, on the other hand, provides a generally complete pattern in any particular system.

The Phosphoglucomutases

There is polymorphic variation at all three of the phosphoglucomutase loci, and this has been investigated in Southern African hunter-gatherer populations for the first and second loci, whose gene products are detectable in red cells, but not for the third, for which nucleated cells are needed. All populations studied to date are polymorphic at the PGM_1 locus; the sample of ‡huã: reported here was too small for it to be stated without reservation that only one allele occurs in the population, though since the sample included most of the surviving ‡huã: this is possible. Frequencies of the commonest variant, PGM_1^2, tend to be low in the Khoisan generally, and lower, on the whole, in the San than in the Khoi (table XVIII). It is possible that the G!ãg!ai as well as the ‡huã: do not possess it, though in the former the rare and interesting PGM_1^6 allele is found. PGM_1^6 occurs in low frequencies in Negro populations, at somewhat higher ones in Mongoloids, and appears in Southern Africa to be associated particularly with the Khoi, in whom its frequency can be as high as or higher than in Chinese and Indonesians. Two individuals, one from Tsumkwe and one among the Hei//om, have been found to possess the even rarer PGM_1^7 variant or one closely resembling it, hitherto only described among the English [HOPKINSON and HARRIS, 1966].

A particular anthropological interest attaches to the second locus, since the PGM_2^2 allele appears possibly to indicate Khoisan descent. Though it has been detected in Negroes from parts of Africa remote from those inhabited by the Khoisan, it reaches much higher frequencies in Southern Africa than anywhere else. Neither the Dama nor the Kwengo, Negro isolates which appear to have received little gene flow from the Khoisan, appear to possess it, and it was not found in the Sesfontein Khoi. The frequencies in the !Xõ, G/wi, G//ana and Hei//om are fairly high, while it was not found in the small ‡huã: and the G!ãg!ai samples and the frequency in the Tsumkwe !Kung is low. The highest frequency of all was somewhat unexpectedly found in the Denasena, whose other gene markers indicate them to be Negro with comparatively little Khoisan admixture. The other, characteristically Negro, variant at this locus, PGM_2^3, seems not to occur in any of these populations.

6-Phosphogluconate Dehydrogenase (6PGD)

It has been pointed out in a recent survey of the distribution of the variants of this enzyme in Southern Africa [JENKINS and NURSE, 1974] that

Table XVIII. Phosphoglucomutase phenotypes and gene frequencies

Population	n		First locus										$\chi^2[1]$	Second locus					$\chi^2[1]$
			phenotypes						gene frequencies					phenotypes			gene frequencies		
			1–1	2–1	2–2	6–1	7–1	6–2, 7–7, etc.	PGM_1^1	PGM_1^2	PGM_1^6	PGM_1^7		1–1	2–1	2–2	PGM_2^1	PGM_2^2	
San																			
G!aokx'ate[10]	33		32	1	0	0	0	0	0.985	0.015	0.000	0.000	0.0	31	2	0	0.970	0.030	0.0
!Xõ[16]	51	obs.	42	7	2	0	0	0	0.856	0.144	0.000	0.000	3.72	46	5	0	0.952	0.048	0.12
		exp.	37.4	12.6	1.1	0	0	0						46.2	4.7	0.1			
ǂhuã[13]	36		36	0	0	0	0	0	1.000	0.000	0.000	0.000		36	0	0	1.000	0.000	
G/wi[7]	93	obs.	67	23	3	0	0	0	0.844	0.156	0.000	0.000	0.31	85	7	1	0.947	0.053	2.23
		exp.	66.2	24.5	2.3	0	0	0						83.4	9.3	0.3			
G//ana[7]	50	obs.	32	18	0	0	0	0	0.820	0.180	0.000	0.000	2.37	47	3	0	0.970	0.030	0.10
		exp.	33.6	14.8	1.6	0	0	0						47.0	2.9	0.1			
Nharo[6]	58		55	3	0	0	0	0	0.974	0.026	0.000	0.000	0.04	54	4	0	0.965	0.035	
//au//en[6]	82		76	6	0	0	0	0	0.963	0.037	0.000	0.000	0.11	78	4	0	0.976	0.024	
!Kung, Dobe[6]	328		315	13	0	0	0	0	0.980	0.020	0.000	0.000	0.11	311	17	0	0.974	0.026	
!Kung, /du/da[6]	74		73	1	0	0	0	0	0.993	0.007	0.000	0.000		69	5	0	0.966	0.034	
!Kung, Tsumkwe[6]	169	obs.	149	15	3	1	1	0	0.906	0.086	0.004	0.004	8.29	167	2	0	0.994	0.006	0.0
		exp.	138.7	26.3	1.2	1.2	1.2	0.4						167.0	2.0	0.0			
!Kung, G!ãg!ai[10]	36		35	0	0	1	0	0	0.986	0.000	0.014	0.000		36	0	0	1.000	0.000	
Khoi																			
Topnaar, Sesfontein[6]	42	obs.	31	7	0	3	0	1	0.856	0.096	0.048	0.000	0.87	42	0	0	1.000	0.000	
		exp.	30.8	6.9	0.4	3.5	0	0.4											
Hei//om[10]	91	obs.	74	15	1	0	1	0	0.901	0.093	0.000	0.006	0.17	81	10	0	0.941	0.059	0.30
		exp.	73.9	15.2	0.8	0	1.0	0.1						80.6	10.1	0.3			
Negro																			
Dama[12]	119	obs.	67	45	7	0	0	0	0.752	0.248	0.000	0.000	0.02	119	0	0	1.000	0.000	
		exp.	67.3	44.4	7.3	0	0	0											
Kwengo[14]	35	obs.	18	16	1	0	0	0	0.743	0.257	0.000	0.000	1.35	35	0	0	1.000	0.000	
		exp.	19.3	13.4	2.3	0	0	0											
Denasena[15]	77	obs.	40	30	7	0	0	0	0.714	0.286	0.000	0.000	0.70	63	13	1	0.903	0.097	
		exp.	39.3	31.4	6.3	0	0	0						62.7	13.5	0.7			

Table XIX. 6PGD phenotypes and gene frequencies

Population	n	Phenotypes					Gene frequencies		
		AA	AC	CC	AR	CR+RR	PGD^A	PGD^C	PGD^R
San									
G!aokx'ate[10]	33	33	0	0	0	0	1.000	0.000	0.000
!Xõ[16]	51	49	2	0	0	0	0.980	0.020	0.000
ǂhuã:[13]	36	36	0	0	0	0	1.000	0.000	0.000
G/wi[7]	94	93	1	0	0	0	0.995	0.005	0.000
G//ana[7]	50	44	6	0	0	0	0.940	0.060	0.000
Nharo[6]	58	57	1	0	0	0	0.991	0.009	0.000
//au//en[6]	82	81	1	0	0	0	0.994	0.006	0.000
!Kung, Dobe[6]	328	328	0	0	0	0	1.000	0.000	0.000
!Kung, /du/da[6]	74	74	0	0	0	0	1.000	0.000	0.000
!Kung, Tsumkwe[6]	147	147	0	0	0	0	1.000	0.000	0.000
!Kung, G!ag!ai[10]	35	35	0	0	0	0	1.000	0.000	0.000
Khoi									
Topnaar, Sesfontein[6]	42	41	0	0	1	0	0.988	0.000	0.012
Hei//om[10]	62	61	1	0	0	0	0.992	0.008	0.000
Negro									
Dama[12]	119	112	4	0	3	0	0.970	0.017	0.013
Kwengo[14]	35	35	0	0	0	0	1.000	0.000	0.000
Denasena[15]	77	73	4	0	0	0	0.974	0.026	0.000

the PGD^C allele is not often present in San populations and, when it is, can be assumed to be an indication of Negro admixture, whereas the PGD^R allele not only has its highest known frequency in the Dama but when it occurs in the adjoining peoples appears to be the result of Dama admixture. This is illustrated by the values in table XIX.

The Peptidases

No clear evidence of polymorphism at either the peptidase B or the peptidase C locus has emerged as yet from the investigation of any Southern African indigenous population, though the occurrence of a 'weak' allele at the peptidase C locus has been suspected. Fairly high frequencies of $PepA^2$ and lower but nevertheless characteristic frequencies of $PepD^2$ tend to occur in the Negro populations; when found in non-Negro peoples, these are useful indications of Negro admixture. It is interesting to note that the suggestion of this in the PGD^c frequency in the G//ana tends to be corroborated by the $PepD^2$ frequency, and that the rather high $PepA^2$ frequency in the ǂhuã:, who are San clients of settled Negro Kgalagadi who probably contribute to their gene pool, is borne out by frequencies of Gd^{A-} and Gd^A high for a San population. Further confirmation is found in the unusually frequent R^2

Table XX. Peptidases A and D phenotypes and gene frequencies

Population	n		Peptidase A					$\chi^2[1]$	Peptidase D							
			phenotypes			gene frequencies			phenotypes					gene frequencies		
			1–1	2–1	2–2	*PepA*[1]	*PepA*[2]		1–1	2–1	2–2	3–1	3–2+3–3	*PepD*[1]	*PepD*[2]	*PepD*[3]
San																
G!aokx'ate[10]	33		33	0	0	1.000	0.000	–	33	0	0	0	0	1.000	0.000	0.000
!Xõ[16]	51		51	0	0	1.000	0.000	–	51	0	0	0	0	1.000	0.000	0.000
ǂhuã[13]	36	obs.	31	4	1	0.917	0.083	3.63	36	0	0	0	0	1.000	0.000	0.000
		exp.	30.3	5.5	0.2											
G/wi[7]	79		78	1	0	0.994	0.006	–	79	0	0	0	0	1.000	0.000	0.000
G//ana[7]	50		49	1	0	0.990	0.010	–	47	3	0	0	0	0.970	0.030	0.000
!Kung, Tsumkwe[6]	278		277	1	0	0.998	0.002	–	276	0	0	0	0	0.996	0.000	0.004
!Kung, G!ãg!ai[10]	35		35	0	0	1.000	0.000	–	35	0	0	0	0	1.000	0.000	0.000
Khoi																
Hei//om[10]	68	obs.	65	2	1	0.967	0.033	9.36	66	0	0	2	0	0.985	0.000	0.015
		exp.	63.6	4.3	0.1											
Negro																
Dama[12]	92		88	4	0	0.978	0.022	–	92	0	0	0	0	1.000	0.000	0.000
Kwengo[14]	35	obs.	29	4	2	0.886	0.114	5.94	35	0	0	0	0	1.000	0.000	0.000
		exp.	27.5	7.1	0.5											
Denasena[15]	77	obs.	72	3	2	0.955	0.045	18.20	77	0	0	0	0	1.000	0.000	0.000
		exp.	70.2	6.6	0.2											

allele in the rhesus system in both the G//ana and the ‡huã:. The *PepD*³ allele found in the Hei//om and the Tsumkwe !Kung, furthermore, attests gene exchanges between these populations already suggested by the presence of PGM_1^7 in both. The Kwengo, who are not in genetic equilibrium for the system, have an exceptionally high frequency of $PepA^2$, which is also worthy of mention. The Denasena and the Hei//om are not in genetic equilibrium either, but do not have a very high frequency of the allele. Neither the Denasena nor the Kwengo show variation in the peptidase D system (table XX).

Acid Phosphatase

Since it has been shown that the P^r allele is almost certainly a Khoisan marker [JENKINS and CORFIELD, 1972], red cell acid phosphatase variation has proved to be of particular interest in African anthropology. In many San populations the frequency of P^r is approximately equal to or even higher than that of P^a, while it is very low in the Dama and much lower in the Kwengo than in any Khoisan population (table XXI). The Hei//om frequency is lower even than that found in the settled Khoi [JENKINS, 1972], while that in the G!aokx'ate is the highest in any known population. Of apparently comparable anthropological importance is the fairly definite demarcation of San populations with a high frequency of P^b from those with a more modest frequency; it is a factor tending to confirm a cline of north-to-south genetic differentiation in the San, which has been mentioned in connection with other systems and will be discussed at greater length later. The very occasional occurrence of an individual bearing the P^c allele may represent the aftermath of gene flow from Caucasoid or, marginally more probably, Mbo sources. It does not seem likely that the P^c of the Mbo is identical with that of Caucasoids [JENKINS *et al.*, in preparation].

Adenylate Kinase

Variation in the adenylate kinase system has as yet been investigated in comparatively few of these hunter-gatherer peoples. All available data are shown in table XXII. The enzyme is probably not polymorphic in Negroes except in Southern and East Africa, and levels of AK^2 as high as those of the Dama, //au//en and Sesfontein Khoi are unusual outside the Indian subcontinent [TILLS *et al.*, 1971]. It becomes very difficult to account for the high Dama frequency except as an extreme example of drift, if the barely polymorphic frequencies in Southern and East African Negroes [JENKINS, 1972] are to be ascribed to Khoisan admixture, as is almost certainly the case in

Table XXI. Erythrocyte acid phosphatase phenotypes and gene frequencies

Population	n		Phenotypes							Gene frequencies				χ^2	d.f.
			AA	AB	BB	AR	BR	RR	all BC+others	P^a	P^b	P^r	P^c		
San															
G!aokx'ate[10]	33	obs.	1	2	7	3	11	9	0	0.106	0.379	0.515		2.60	3
		exp.	0.4	2.7	4.7	3.6	12.9	8.7	0						
!Xõ[16]	51	obs.	12	14	8	5	8	4	0	0.422	0.372	0.206		4.48	3
		exp.	9.1	16.0	7.1	8.9	7.8	2.2	0.0						
ǂhuã:[13]	35	obs.	2	10	5	5	11	2	0	0.271	0.443	0.286		1.77	3
		exp.	2.6	8.4	6.9	5.4	8.9	2.9	0						
G/wi[7]	94	obs.	11	18	13	15	25	10	2	0.292	0.367	0.331	0.010	2.10	3
		exp.	8.0	20.1	12.7	18.2	22.8	10.3	1.9						
G//ana[7]	49	obs.	13	10	6	10	7	3	0	0.469	0.296	0.235		2.17	2
		exp.	10.8	13.6	4.3	10.8	6.8	2.7	0						
Nharo[6]	36	obs.	3	8	12	1	8	4	0	0.208	0.556	0.236		5.43	3
		exp.	1.6	8.3	11.1	3.5	9.4	2.0	0						
!Kung, Tsumkwe[6]	271	obs.	17	45	101	31	64	13	0	0.203	0.574	0.223		10.42	3
		exp.	11.2	63.2	89.3	24.5	69.4	13.5	0						
!Kung, G!ãg!ai[10]	36	obs.	1	7	15	6	5	2	0	0.208	0.538	0.208		5.48	3
		exp.	1.6	8.7	12.2	3.1	8.7	1.6	0						
Khoi															
Hei//om[10]	69	obs.	6	14	29	8	10	2	0	0.246	0.594	0.159		5.55	3
		exp.	4.2	20.2	24.3	5.4	13.0	1.7	0						
Negro															
Dama[12]	92	obs.	2	30	58	0	1	0	1	0.190	0.799	0.005	0.006	0.66	1
		exp.	3.3	27.9	58.7	0.2	0.7	0.0	1.1						
Kwengo[14]	35	obs.	2	17	11	1	3	1	0	0.314	0.600	0.086		4.54	3
		exp.	3.5	13.2	12.6	1.9	3.6	0.3	0						
Denasena[15]	77	obs.	3	16	51	0	6	1	0	0.143	0.805	0.052		5.74	3
		exp.	1.6	17.7	49.9	1.1	6.4	0.2	0						

Table XXII. Adenylate kinase phenotypes and gene frequencies

Population	n		Phenotypes			Gene frequencies		χ^2[1]
			1–1	2–1	2–2	AK^1	AK^2	
San								
G!aokx'ate[10]	33	obs.	33	0	0	1.000	0.000	0.00
		exp.	–	–	–			
Nharo[6]	58	obs.	50	8	0	0.931	0.069	0.33
		exp.	50.2	7.5	0.3			
//au//en[6]	82	obs.	68	14	0	0.915	0.085	0.72
		exp.	68.6	12.8	0.6			
!Kung, Dobe[6]	328	obs.	312	16	0	0.976	0.024	0.22
		exp.	312.4	15.4	0.2			
!Kung, /du/da[6]	74	obs.	63	10	1	0.919	0.081	0.59
		exp.	62.5	11.0	0.5			
!Kung, Tsumkwe[6]	147	obs.	131	16	0	0.946	0.054	0.47
		exp.	131.6	15.0	0.4			
Khoi								
Topnaar, Sesfontein[6]	42	obs.	34	8	0	0.905	0.095	0.49
		exp.	34.4	7.2	0.4			
Hei//om[10]	51	obs.	47	4	0	0.960	0.040	0.10
		exp.	47.0	3.9	0.1			
Negro								
Dama[12]	119	obs.	98	21	0	0.912	0.088	1.10
		exp.	99.0	19.1	0.9			
Denasena[15]	77	obs.	77	0	0	1.000	0.000	0.00
		exp.	–	–	–			

the Cape Coloureds [Gordon *et al.*, 1966]. It will be obvious from most of the tables that the Khoisan genetic contribution to the Dama has been slight. On the other hand, the Dama have made an appreciable contribution to the gene pools of their neighbours and erstwhile masters [Nurse *et al.*, 1976]. Until it is possible to establish whether or not the Dama AK^2 and the Khoisan AK^2 are responsible for chemically as well as electrophoretically identical gene products, this question will remain unsettled.

Other Enzyme Polymorphisms

Botha *et al.* [1973] report that 59–73 individuals from the Tsumkwe !Kung were tested for variation in the lactate dehydrogenase A and B, isocitrate dehydrogenase, phosphoglycerate kinase and malate dehydrogenase systems without the detection of any variant. Esterase D has been investigated in the !Xõ (five 2–1 heterozygotes in a population sample of 51, gene frequency $EsD^2 = 0.049$), the ǂhuã: (1 out of 35, $EsD^2 = 0.014$), the G!aokx'ate (no variation in 33) and the Denasena (3 out of 77, $EsD^2 = 0.020$). Carbonic anhydrases I and II, isocitrate dehydrogenase and glutathione peroxidase have been investigated only in the G!aokx'ate and the Denasena. The G!aokx'ate showed no variation in any of these systems, and the Denasena were uniformly CA_1 1 but in 77 individuals revealed 9 who were CA_{11} 2–1 ($CA_{11}{}^2$ = 0.058) and 2 who were ICD 4–1 (ICD^4 = 0.013). There were also 11 Denasena with the fast variant of glutathione peroxidase, the mode of inheritance of which is uncertain. The same two populations have been investigated for variation in the glutamyl pyruvate transaminase system. Five G!aokx'ate were GPT 1, 20 were GPT 2–1 and 8 GPT 2, giving a Gpt^2 frequency of 0.546 and generating $\chi^2_{[1]}$ of 1.60. Among the Denasena, 56 were GPT 1, 19 GPT 2–1 and 1 GPT 2, with Gpt^2 frequency of 0.149 and $\chi^2_{[1]}$ of 0.07.

Serum Protein Polymorphisms

The Gm System

JENKINS and STEINBERG [1966], JENKINS *et al.* [1970] and JENKINS and BRAIN [1967] have reported extensively on Gm patterns in hunter-gatherers in Southern Africa, and further data are given in STEINBERG *et al.* [1975]; these are presented in tables XXIIIa and b. It will be seen that in three !Kung populations and the //au//en the unusual $Gm^{1,5,13,14,21}$ haplotype occurs, reaching quite a high frequency in the Dobe !Kung. The $Gm^{1,5}$ haplotype is found in the Nharo, //au//en and northern and Ngami !Kung, though at rather low frequencies. The commonest haplotype in the San is $Gm^{1,13}$, and they also possess the $Gm^{1,21}$ haplotype in fairly high frequencies. Though the Khoi $Gm^{1,13}$ frequency is also quite high, they do not seem to have $Gm^{1,21}$ but to possess $Gm^{1,2,21}$, which is absent from the San. None of these haplotypes was found in the very small sample of Dama who, however, share with both San and Khoi, and with all Negro populations so far investigated, the characteristically African $Gm^{1,5,13,14}$ haplotype. The more specifically Negro haplotypes $Gm^{1,5,6}$ and $Gm^{1,5,6,14}$, and the $Gm^{1,5,14}$ which, despite its apparent association with Negroes, reaches its highest known frequencies in a population of settled Khoi and a mixed Khoi/Caucasoid population without

---

Fig. 8. The $Gm^{1,21}$ and $Gm^{1,2,21}$ alleles appear to distinguish fairly sharply between San and Khoi. One would not expect to find either in the unmixed Negroes, such as the Dama shown here.

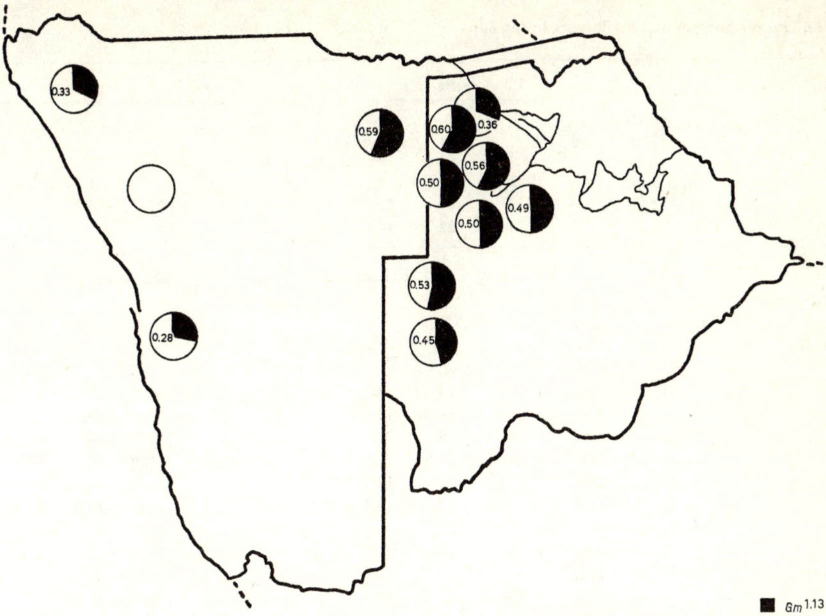

Fig. 7. The distribution of the $Gm^{1,\ 13}$ allele, showing high frequencies in the San, moderate frequencies in the Khoi, and apparent absence from the only virtually unmixed Negro population so far tested for this system.

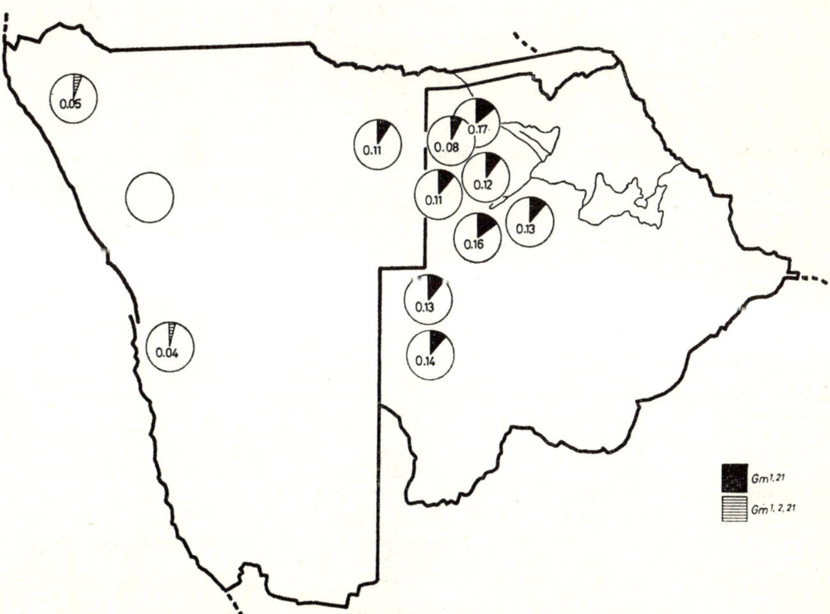

Table XXIIIa. Gm phenotypes and haplotypes in the San

Population	n		Phenotypes 1 5 13 14	1 5 13 14 21	1 5 6 13 14	1 5 6 13 14 21	1 5 6 14	1 5 6 14 21	1 13	1 13 21	1 5 6 13	1 5 6 21	
San													
Southern + Central[6]	112	obs.	57		5		2		38		0		2
		exp.	56.9		5.3		1.8		36.0		1.2		0
Southern, mainly, !Xõ[6]	72	obs.	30		14		2		23		1		0
		exp.	30.6		12.4		3.2		23.5		0.8		0
Nharo[6]	138	obs.	46	14	13	0	0	2	40	18	2	1	
		exp.	49.6	10.0	12.1	0	0.6	1.8	38.1	19.5	2.2	0.6	
//au//en[6]	258	obs.	86	29	21	0	1	0	62	44	0	1	
		exp.	88.2	27.6	17.1	0.3	1.1	3.3	64.3	40.0	1.7	0.5	
!Kung, northern[6]	100	obs.	26	30	12	0	0	4	13	12	0	0	
		exp.	27.6	27.6	10.2	1.7	0.8	2.7	13.3	12.4	0	0	
!Kung, Ngami[6]	152	obs.	52	20	6	0	1	0	32	23	3	0	
		exp.	52.6	19.3	5.5	0.6	0.5	0.7	36.3	18.8	2.1	0.6	
!Kung, Dobe[6]	394	obs.	155	33	19	0	0	1	142	40	2	0	
		exp.	156.0	32.1	17.5	0.4	0.3	1.6	143.1	38.6	1.7	0.2	
!Kung, /ai/ai[6]	62	obs.	33	4	2	0	0	0	16	5	0	0	
		exp.	32.4	4.9	1.8	0.0	0.0	0.2	15.5	6.5	0	0	
!Kung, /du/da[6]	100	obs.	38	11	6	0	0	0	33	11	0	0	
		exp.	41.5	7.1	5.1	0.0	0.1	0.7	30.8	13.3	0	0	
!Kung, Tsumkwe[6]	197	obs.	77	13	1	0	0	0	74	17	6	0	
		exp.	79.4	10.0	1.6	0.0	0.3	0.0	69.4	26.1	4.2	0.8	

Table XXIIIb. Gm phenotypes and haplotypes in the Khoi and Negroes

Population	n		Phnntxpes 1 5 13 14	1 5 13 14 21	1 5 6 13 14	1 5 6 13 14 21	1 5 6 14	1 5 6 14 21	1 13	1 13 21	1 5 6 13	1 5 6 21	
Khoi													
Topnaar, Kuiseb[6]	57	obs.	16		23		5		5		1		0
		exp.	16.4		21		5.9		4.4		1.4		0
Topnaar, Sesfontein[6]	42	obs.	20	0	12	0	1	0	4	0	1	0	
		exp.	19.7	0	11.4	0	1.5	0	4.6	0	0.8	0.0	
Negro													
Dama[6]	25	obs.	9		13		2		0		0		1
		exp.	9.0		12.0		2.6		0		0		1

					Haplotypes								χ²	d.f.
1 5 14 21	1 21	1 5 21	1 5	1 5 13	1 5 13 14	1 5 13 14 21	1 13	1 21	1 5 6 14	1 5	1 5 6	1 5 14		
	4	3		1	0.317		0.384	0.227	0.024	0.030	0.014	0.000	3.30	2
	5.8	1.7		2.6										
	2	0		0	0.290		0.452	0.135	0.111	0.000	0.012	0.000	1.70	1
	1.3	0		0										
0	1	0	0	1	0.270	0.000	0.526	0.134	0.050	0.005	0.015	0.000	3.06	3
0	2.5	0.2	0.0	0.7										
0	6	0	0	7	0.262	0.014	0.499	0.155	0.041	0.022	0.006	0.000	9.37	5
0	6.2	1.8	0.1	5.7										
0	2	0	0	1	0.272	0.106	0.364	0.170	0.080	0.008	0.000	0.000	3.46	3
0	2.9	0.3	0.0	0.6										
0	2	0	0	13	0.254	0.033	0.489	0.126	0.019	0.063	0.014	0.000	7.63	4
0	2.4	2.4	0.6	9.4										
0	2	0	0	0	0.268	0.020	0.603	0.081	0.024	0.000	0.004	0.000	1.34	2
0	2.6	0	0	0										
0	2	0	0	0	0.378	0.000	0.501	0.105	0.016	0.000	0.000	0.000	1.22	1
0	0.7	0	0	0										
0	1	0	0	0	0.295	0.000	0.555	0.120	0.030	0.000	0.000	0.000	3.87	2
0	1.4	0	0	0										
4	5	0	0	0	0.227	0.000	0.593	0.112	0.000	0.000	0.018	0.050	11.31	4
2.2	2.4	0	0	0										

								Haplotypes						χ²	d.f.
1 2 3 1	1 2 5 13 14 (21)	1 2 5 6 (21)	1 2 5 6 14 (21)	1 2 3 5 13 14 (21)	1 3 5 13 14	1 3 5 6 13 14	3 5 13 14	1 5 13 14	1 5 13 14 21	1 13	1 5 6 14	1 5 6	1 2 21	3 5 13 14		
	1	1	2	0	2	0	1	0.330		0.280	0.280	0.040	0.040	0.040	2.73	5
.1	1.3	0.2	1.1	0.1	2.4	1.3	0.1									
	1	0	1	0	0	0	0	0.429	0.000	0.333	0.163	0.027	0.048	0.000	0.94	2
.3	1.7	0	0.6	0	0	0	0									
	0	0	0	0	0	0	0	0.601		0.000	0.166	0.233	0.000	0.000	0.15	1
	0	0	0	0	0	0	0									

other evidence of a Negro contribution, are all found in these desert-dwellers but in an unrevealing distribution. Of the three, $Gm^{1,5,6,14}$ is the commonest and is found in all the populations except the Tsumkwe !Kung; it occurs at fairly high frequency in the two Khoi populations and the Dama. $Gm^{1,5,6}$ appears to be a more reliable indicator of Negro contribution; its frequency in the Dama is high, while it is absent from the northern !Kung and those of /ai/ai and /du/da, is at low frequencies in the other San populations and is slightly more common in the Khoi. Though $Gm^{1,2,21}$ is probably found in unmixed Khoi populations, $Gm^{3,5,13,14}$ is certainly an indication of Caucasoid admixture with the Kuiseb Khoi.

This system appears to be one of the most useful so far discovered for the elucidation of anthropological problems, though it sometimes poses further problems which demand more material.

The Inv System

By contrast with Gm, the Inv system is of very little anthropological value. The range of Inv^1 frequencies in hunter-gatherer populations is comprehended in the wider Southern African range; the only exception is in the Kuiseb Khoi, whose very high frequency could be ascribed to the Caucasoid admixture which is known to have taken place or to the inclusion of a number of related individuals. The latter could also be the reason for the tendency of most of these frequencies among hunter-gatherers to lie at or towards the lower end of the range. The figures are shown in table XXIV.

Table XXIV. Inv phenotypes and gene frequencies

Population	n	Phenotypes		Gene frequencies	
		Inv(1+)	Inv(1–)	$Inv^1 + Inv^{1,2}$	Inv^3
San					
Southern and Central	112	62	50	0.331	0.669
Southern, mainly !Xo[6]	72	37	35	0.303	0.697
Nharo[6]	140	82	58	0.357	0.643
//au//en[6]	263	150	113	0.344	0.656
!Kung, northern[6]	103	62	41	0.369	0.631
!Kung, Ngami[6]	156	97	59	0.385	0.615
!Kung, Dobe[6]	394	253	141	0.402	0.598
!Kung, /ai/ai[6]	62	35	27	0.340	0.660
!Kung, /du/da[6]	100	60	40	0.367	0.633
!Kung, Tsumkwe[6]	198	136	62	0.440	0.560
Khoi					
Topnaar, Kuiseb[6]	57	17	40	0.162	0.838
Topnaar, Sesfontein[6]	42	25	17	0.364	0.636

The Pseudocholinesterase C_5 Polymorphism

Very little is known about the genetics of the variation occurring in this system, and only four populations have been investigated for it. The C_5 (+) phenotype appears to be unusually common among the Dama and the Dobe !Kung; but the significance of this cannot be determined until much more material is available. None of the 57 Kuiseb Topnaar was C_5 (+), but among the 40 Sesfontein Topnaar examined there was 1 positive. This may be due to a contribution to the gene pool by the Dama, who showed 6 positives out of 91. The frequency among the Dobe !Kung was almost as high, with 5 positives out of 98. It will be interesting to see whether this trend is confirmed when further San populations are examined.

Chromosome Studies

It is perhaps not surprising that there should as yet have been few chromosomes studies on Southern African hunter-gatherers. WALLACE and HALLET [personal commun., 1974] have examined the karyotypes of 3 female and 5 male !Kung, and noticed nothing out of the ordinary in comparison with the karyotypes of Caucasoid or Negroid South Africans. Cytogenetic studies carried out on Khoi not, admittedly, hunter-gatherers, by HELTNE and SINGER [1971] showed unexpected results. They found a high percentage of aneuploid cells; the rate increased with age and was significantly higher than for any other population. A small fragment of chromatin was found in the two Khoi males and in 22 of the 23 females studied. The significance of such a finding is not apparent but the authors suggest it may result from hybridization between Khoi, on the one hand, and San or Negroes, on the other.

Chapter 5. Adaptation to the Environment

A great variety of factors, far greater than have yet been investigated, are involved in any biological adaptive situation, and those which do come to be investigated tend to represent the individual interests of particular workers. The San occupy a special place in the social mythology of South African Caucasoids, and the conviction that they are unique and remarkable has led to their being more variously, though not necessarily more thoroughly, studied than many more accessible and not less interesting peoples. Luckily, the 'River Bushmen', represented in this review by the Kwengo, are generally subsumed into the myth as San, and have had a little more attention paid to them than might have been the case had they been recognized as being Negro.

Three exogenous or environmental categories of adaptation have been studied in certain of these hunter-gatherer groups. Those that dwell in deserts have been particularly favoured for such studies, and in most deserts there are considerable diurnal and seasonal variations in the ambient temperature. The relevance of these to the adaptation of certain San groups and one group of Kwengo has been investigated. The nutritional status of hunter-gatherers has interested a number of workers, and those in Southern Africa have perhaps received more attention than many others. Exogenous disease, whether due to environmental trauma or to the operation of infective agents, is obviously important, though the studies here have not been extensive.

Closely linked to nutrition, and of great adaptive significance, are the questions of growth and physique and of the metabolic peculiarities of these peoples. It is known that a considerable corpus of data exists on these subjects, though a comparatively small proportion has been published. The accounts of inherited disorders in these populations are as yet sparse and are probably limited by social factors to be discussed below.

The question of the psychological adjustment of hunter-gatherers to the environment is, as REUNING and WORTLEY [1973] point out, of no more and no less interest than that of the adjustment any human groups to any circumstances familiar to them but not to the investigator. Hunter-gatherers, like farmers and city-dwellers, are subjected to a finite range of stimuli, and their responses are limited to those of which any human animals are capable. It is mainly in order to determine the general range of human capacity to respond that psychological studies of such extreme populations are of value.

Temperature Adjustment

Two questions are presented by the extremes of temperature found in deserts: that of the degree to which the inhabitants are unaffected by cold, and the extent and nature of their acclimatization to heat. The survival of the desert-dwellers virtually unclothed in conditions of both extreme cold and extreme heat might suggest that some form of tolerance of fluctuations in temperature could constitute a factor in their adaptation. The degree of such adaptation has been studied for the San in a series of well-controlled experiments conducted by WYNDHAM and co-workers. They found [WYNDHAM and MORRISON, 1956; WYNDHAM *et al.*, 1964b] that the responses of the San to heat, as measured by heart rate, are better than those of both unacclimatized Caucasoids and unacclimatized Negroes. In contrast, the Kwengo showed similarities in their heart rates to those developed by acclimatized Negroes but lower than those of unacclimatized Negroes. The rectal temperatures of both are between those of unacclimatized Caucasoids and Negroes. Both the San and the Kwengo do, however, show unequivocal signs of acclimatization to heat in their sweat rates, which are about midway between those of acclimatized and unacclimatized men.

It must be borne in mind that the criteria of acclimatization to heat adopted by WYNDHAM and his team are particularly rigorous. They relate not simply to residence in a hot climate, but to the ability to perform arduous physical labour under conditions of high ambient temperature. It is rarely necessary for a Southern African hunter-gatherer to subject himself to such extreme discomfort. The energy expenditure of 5 kcal/min while hunting, which is that estimated by WYNDHAM for the San, is, as he says, a moderate rate of work, but there is no firm evidence of the length of time for which it is uninterruptedly sustained. The contrast of the success of the San in the chase with his comparatively poor performance in the climatic tent suggests that guile is probably more important than physique in his adaptation to his environment.

This view is reinforced by the findings of WYNDHAM and his team in their studies of the adjustment to cold of the Kalahari San [WYNDHAM and MORRISON, 1958; WARD *et al.*, 1960; WYNDHAM *et al.*, 1964a]. They found that the air temperature under the skin cloak of the sleeping San on a winter night was about 26 °C, though that near the extremities it was somewhat lower. They point out that the San has succeeded by intellectual rather than physiological adaptation in producing for himself during the coldest part of the day a microclimate which is approximately in the thermoneutral zone. Deliberate exposure to cold evoked a greater fall in rectal temperature than was found in Caucasoids, though no greater than that of Negroes. WYNDHAM interprets this as a reaction to less adequate insulation by subcutaneous tissues rather than as thermal adaptation.

Endurance Capacity

Endurance capacity, like temperature adjustment, relates to the work performed by hunter-gatherers in securing subsistence. Intrinsic to the mythology cherished by the South African Caucasoid about the San is the image of the tireless pursuer of a wounded animal, the little man who can outpace his kill. That this is a myth was indicated by *ad hoc* tests carried out by BRONTË-STEWART *et al.* [1960] and has been clearly demonstrated by STRYDOM [1973].

Endurance capacity is determined by the ability of an individual's cardiorespiratory and muscular systems to extract and use the oxygen in the inspired air. This ability is measured by the maximum oxygen intake test; oxygen intake and heart rate during exercise are plotted against each other and straight line extrapolation taken to a standard maximum, usually a heart rate of 180/min. STRYDOM performed the test in the field on 24 San males of unspecified groups, and found that their endurance capacities were on average very much lower than those of Caucasoid and Negro athletes, appreciably lower than those of Negro labourers and Caucasoid army recruits, and approximately equal to those of a rather sedentary group of medical students. Only two men in his sample had endurance capacities suggesting an ability to perform as well as unexceptional middle-distance runners. STRYDOM, too, makes the point that their adaptation 'must be attributed not to their physical or physiological potentialities but to their wit'.

Social Adjustment

The basic pressure regulating social adjustment among hunter-gatherers, as among all other peoples, is that exerted by the environment. The individual may be able to survive, and the nuclear family to reproduce itself, but the group by exploiting variation in the talents and abilities of its members will make a more effective and economical use of resources and prove more resistant to natural stresses. This imposes the ethological imperative of the development of sets of within-group signs by means of which cooperative communication can take place [KUMMER, 1969]. It has been suggested by EIBL-EIBESFELDT [1969] that there is a phylogenetic, i.e. inherited, component in social adaptation, but that behavioural resemblances among distantly related species may be due to parallel evolution in analogous environments. He stresses the similarities in social behaviour among all human groups so far studied, and makes the telling point [EIBL-EIBESFELDT, 1972] that many such similarities are now functionally neutral and may represent relics of some earlier stage.

WILMSEN [1973] has considered the organization of hunter-gatherer groups as a special case of more general interaction and spacing processes. He points out that if food resources are concentrated and shifting, as they are for the Southern African hunter-gatherers, it is more efficient if group exploitation is carried out by central localization of the population. This seems to mean that a migrant band would ideally follow a cyclical path describing a perimeter of which the radius would be equal to the radius of possible exploitation. This would, of course, only be the case where the cycle of availability of resources operated at a constant rate and all concentrations were of equal utility; in practice in Southern Africa this is not so, and migration paths are both temporally and spatially irregular. Consequently, the assertion of territoriality is moderated by overlaps at particular concentrations of resources in excess of the requirements of any one band and tends to be extended where resources are sparser.

Coming to the internal organization of the band, WILMSEN [1973] states that: 'The most stable identifiable units in this structure are (1) the band itself, (2) the household-residence unit composed of one or more nuclear families plus extensions and (3) the task group composed of active adults drawn from these households.' The band is limited in size by the balance between the resources and the requirements of procurement roles, often by a dispersion of gatherers to maximize the return from stable resources and a concentration of hunters more effectively to deal with mobile game. Since no resource is uniformly abundant, resource roles need to be recombined as necessary to cope with divergent situations.

Stability of the band is maintained by reciprocity conventions among the kinships which comprise it. These have been described by MARSHALL [1961] for the !Kung San of north-western Botswana. Social tensions are relieved by extensive and patient discussion of any point likely to lead to discord, by the elaboration of jokes, by sharing of consumer goods, especially meat and tobacco, and by the giving of gifts to avert jealousy and promote goodwill. Much the same mechanisms are described by HEINZ [1967] for the !Xõ. There is no clear social stratification except in particular circumstances; a good hunter will lead in the hunt, but relinquish the control of weapon-making to a superior craftsman [TANAKA, 1969]. Similar checks tending towards internal social stability are described by KNUSSMANN [1969] for the Dama. Restraint in eating is an aspect of good manners among the !Kung, and so is the avoidance of the giving of offence. Joking relationships, often based on kinship or quasi-kinship, facilitate frank but licensed criticism; resentment or loss of temper signalizes breakdown of this release mechanism, and leads to ostracism. Despite the fact that life is largely conducted in public, individual and sub-group privacy is respected. Gossip is spread only among kinships and intimates; when it becomes general it is seen as disruptive, and avoided.

Hunter-gatherer kinship systems tend to be limited both by generation length and by band size. It is rare to find more than three generations alive in one band at one time, and the linking presence of the common ancestor is the main stimulus to a sense of kinship. SILBERBAUER [1965], who has investigated kinship among the G/wi, points out that for the individual this means that the kin group extends during the course of the life span through the two ascending to the two descending generations. Relationship is recognized both matrilaterally and patrilaterally by most San groups, though large extended agnatic kinships characterize the Dama [VEDDER, 1923]. The principle of avoidance of proximate and the linking of alternate generations necessarily holds, as it does in any system the members of which are in close and frequent contact. As in most such systems, a network of classification defines the members of a kin group in relation to each individual, and there is a rigid demarcation between affinal and cognate kin. There is birth order hierarchy among siblings, and among half-siblings hierarchy depends on the relative seniority of the parents not in common. As in most classificatory systems, the rôle transcends the individual, and biological and recognized forms of relationship often do not coincide. The stability of the kin group is maintained by precise recognition of the degree of familiarity which can be shown by any member towards any other member, and by definition of the duties implicit in any particular bond.

Households may be monogamous or, more rarely, polygamous. Temperamental incompatibility between spouses, or actual or imminent adultery, threatens concord in the band and leads to easy divorce. Households consequently often consist of a married couple and children belonging to the father or mother only. The widowed or divorced reconstitute households by fairly frequent remarriage. The elderly in a preliterate society are the custodians of tradition and experience, are highly regarded and frequently constitute focal points for intrafamilial bonding. SILBERBAUER [1965] was unable to find any evidence to support the belief, common among South African Caucasoids, that the San abandon their aged, but TANAKA [personal commun., 1972] knows of one case where a sick woman was abandoned by her husband who was anxious for the safety of their children.

Another myth, popularized to some extent by THOMAS [1959], claims that the San are completely unaggressive. There is certainly active social discouragement of within-group aggression, but the relationships between bands are often marked by fear and disapproval [MARSHALL, 1959]. In times of shortage particularly, territoriality is aggressively maintained, and fights between bands may lead to realignments of band memberships and reapportionment of territories. If hunting or gathering is to be carried out in the territory of another band, it is customary to seek the permission of that band first. Among the !Kung good manners require that on the approach of strangers all the men should lay down their arms and approach one another unarmed [MARSHALL, 1961]. The tribes of the central Kalahari maintain a system of band alliances, of varying strengths and obscure origin [SILBERBAUER, 1965], which facilitate the exchange of members and marriage partners.

Another form of between-group social adjustment is that which subsists in the clientage relationship of the ǂhuã: with certain Kgalagadi villages, of some of the !Kung, //au//en and Nharo and most of the G!aokx'ate with Herero, of the Denasena of north-eastern Botswana with Kalang'a and Mangwato, and of some groups of Kgalagadi with the Ngwaketse [SCHAPERA, 1953]. At one time, this amounted to virtual serfdom, with the hunting and gathering skills of the serf exerted mainly for the benefit of the master without any recourse to the legal system under which the master lived. Nowadays, however, the relationship persists on a basis which is either voluntary or habitual, without coercion and to the mutual benefit of the parties. It seems to function principally as a means of exchange of manufactured goods for natural products, mainly meat, and services, and could be construed as a mercantile rather than a social relationship, and hence on a par with the San settlements of the farms of Caucasoids. There is no doubt, however, that the patrons do act in many cases as intermediaries between the hunter-gatherers and outsider groups, and thus in their turn help to lessen the tensions of the hunter-gatherer's life.

The Psychology of Hunter-Gatherers

Viewed in the light of the adaptation of hunter-gatherers to the environment, a rather formal approach to their psychology is called for; this has been provided by REUNING and WORTLEY [1973] and REUNING [1973] for the San and to a lesser extent by KNUSSMANN [1969] for the Dama. Earlier accounts of the subject are anecdotal and confusing, and range from high commendation of adaptive learning skills to condemnation of superstition and degraded morals. The picturesque horror of ALEXANDER [1838], when with charming hospitality a party of 'Boschmen' invited him and his men to make free with their wives, has to be read about in his own words to be credited. Yet CHAPMAN [1971], a far more experienced traveller of the 1860s, though occasionally shocked by what he regarded as a taste for squalor, made ready use of San guides for taking his animals safely and efficiently through the tsetse belt of northern Botswana. DORNAN [1922] gives a good unadorned but also unanalytic account of the adaptive value of certain affective and cognitive traits in the San, Denasena and Kgalagadi; he regards the last-named as less skilled in hunting than the two former, whose abilities he puts about equal. His account of their 'mental life' is concerned mostly with folk-tales.

Neither in his major description of the Dama (1923) nor in his subsequent supplement to it (1965) did VEDDER venture to advance any theory about the psychology of the Dama, and KNUSSMANN [1969] seems determined to emphasize their child-like and passive qualities and incapacity for numerical ratiocination. He does, however, point out that they are eager for schooling, and it is perhaps among the schoolchildren of this generation, the adults of the next, that the most culture-free assessment of these people might be obtained.

The investigations of REUNING [1973] and REUNING and WORTLEY [1973] were carried out on Nharo, G/wi and G//ana, and probably some //au//en as well, at Caucasoid-owned farms and cattleposts in the Ghanzi area of western Botswana; on G/wi and G//ana near ǂKade Pan in the Central Kalahari, populations probably identical with the G/wi and G//ana of the serogenetic sample [JENKINS *et al.*, 1975]; on the !Xõ to the south of Ghanziland, populations represented also by the samples described by JENKINS *et al.* [1968] and that for which more extended genetic marker studies are reported for the first time in this monograph; and on a population near Motokwe which was in all probability ǂhuã:.

REUNING and WORTLEY [1973] initiated their project by adapting existing tests and constructing new ones for the assessment of the cognitive functions and, if possible, other psychological traits of the San. Communication limitations required that they should confine themselves to non-verbal performance tests and to experiments which could be conducted with a minimum of verbal explanation. The tests were presented as 'games', and there is evidence that the subjects found the procedures enjoyable. *Sand drawing* was used to explore the pictorial abilities of the San, in the light of the strange fact that the modern San, unlike their ancestors, do not make pictures on the walls of caves. *Symmetry completion, object relations* and *size constancy* tests provided an array of mutually complementary methods of assessing cognitive function. Further tests of learning, visual acuity, manual dexterity, speed and accuracy of perception, temperament in work behaviour, interests and aesthetic preferences were also carried out.

The investigators found that their test scores, estimated by correlating the scores of parts of the tests, were satisfactorily reliable. They interpret this as signifying that the differences between individuals were so great that even comparatively crude techniques would have been able to measure them. Variances among the San were as large as or larger than those found in other groups. This was unexpected, considering that the environments of the populations studied were apparently much less heterogeneous than those of most other populations. The specific effects of contact with Negro and Caucasoid groups seemed to consist mostly in enhancing speed of work and the richness of content in the drawings. They state that: 'It is an open question whether the moderate correlations between performances on some tests and amount of culture contact indicate an effect of the latter, or whether those Bushmen who are alert and able seek more culture contact.' The vision and hearing of the San were equal or superior to those of Caucasoids and Negroes. The 'range of uncertainty' in the size constancy test was smaller than in other groups, and the scores were higher, even in the women whose daily activities do not require such skills; this suggested a genetic factor operating under selective pressure. The results of the object relations test, however, yielded poor scores on average though the range of the scores was wide. This test appears to be more dependent than other assays of cognition are on environmental restrictions. In symmetry completion, the pattern completion part of the test produced high scores, while rotational symmetry completion results seemed to be more influenced by previous cultural contact with outsiders.

The authors conclude that the capacity for conceptual abstraction and the formulation of general principles is relatively undeveloped or 'latent' in the San on account of the cultural lack of any necessity for such a capacity. Despite the minimal amount of specialized training available to them, the San do, however, manifest a 'general intelligence' factor of fair flexibility, and one which does not reduce their ability to adapt to novel and unfamiliar problem situations. 'Lack of formal training in specific fields of knowledge does not appear to lead, necessarily, to an undifferentiated uniformity of approach to a variety of new problems.' They could find no indications of any mental shortcomings in the San, nor did their results suggest that these populations differed in any marked way from other human groups. They emphasize, however, that more specific and detailed studies are called for, particularly in fields where psychological studies could interact with other disciplines such as linguistics or social anthropology.

These findings can be supplemented by the results of electroencephalogram studies carried out by Van Wyk [1964] and Nelson [1964]. The San were found to have a significantly higher alpha frequency (10.6 ± 1.08 cps) than either Negroes or Caucasoids, suggesting a higher average psychic tempo. This may be related to their hunting and gathering pursuits and consequent dependence on visual perception. Nelson [1964] suggests that the more occipital alpha rhythm in the San and the absence of such EEG abnormalities as beta or theta waves indicate that the San have a less emotional and perhaps more intellectual approach than Negroes. Reuning and Wortley [1973] were nevertheless unable to correlate the EEG results with their findings, and the exact significance of such contrasts remains uncertain.

We have not been able to find any account of mental illness in any of the hunter-gatherer populations of Southern Africa, unless the well-attested 'trance state' of the San, observed independently by both of us and described verbally and in print by many of our informants, may be taken as a sign of mental aberration. The practice of going into a trance as part of a process of divination is nonetheless common to a wide variety of cultures, including several Western sub-cultures and, though its precise psychological components remain obscure, it would be presumptuous to describe it as an abnormality. Reliable accounts of it may be found for the G/wi in SILBERBAUER [1965] and for the !Kung in MARSHALL [1962]. It occurs as part of a 'curing dance', and is confined to men who have received instruction in 'curing'. The main difference from its occurrence in other populations consists in the fact that such men comprise all or almost all the mature male members of the band.

Diet and Nutritional Status

KNUSSMANN [1969], in his extremely wide-ranging study of the Dama, passes over the question of their nutritional habits and status with a brief reference to the contrast between the slenderness of the men an the sturdiness of the women. He states that their standard of nutrition 'lies within normal limits'. The present writers are unable to add more than anecdotal details to this: where the Dama do not have herds they hunt the game to be found in the neighbourhood of the Brandberg. Of the gathered food most appears to be varieties of corms and bulbs, described under the blanket term *uientjies,* little onions. Malnutrition, if it occurs, appears to be rare among the Dama, though KÖHLER [1959] mentions that the diet of those living to the west of the Brandberg can be meagre.

VAN WARMELO [1962] describes the inhabitants of the Kaokoveld as 'in dietetic equilibrium with their environment'. McCALMAN and GROBBELAAR [1965] state that Cimba men hunt antelopes but prefer zebra meat to all other; they also gather honey, but the rest of the gathering of 'numerous varieties of edible plants' is done by the women. The specifically nutritional survey conducted by VAN DER MERWE [1969a] concluded that their intake of animal protein was sparse and irregular, and that wild vegetables formed the greater part of their diet. He found that their skinfold thicknesses differed very little from those of their pastoralist neighbours the Himba, and that their nutritional status was very similar.

JENKINS and BRAIN [1967] found no evidence of malnutrition in the Topnaar of the Kuiseb Valley, and JENKINS [personal observation] found no overt signs of it among those in Sesfontein. Nothing seems to have been recorded about the dietary habits or nutritional status of the Hei//om, but they are unlikely to differ from those of other hunter-gatherer peoples of the region.

As might be expected, a number of San groups have been investigated in this connection. BRONTË-STEWART *et al.* [1960] have published an account of their findings in the !Kung of the Kavango area, members of the same or similar groups as the G!ãg!ai mentioned in the serogenetic section. They report a shortage of game in the area and state that the sources of protein were mostly insects and plants, particularly the nuts of the *mangeti* tree, *Ricinodendron rautanenii*. Depending on the availability of foodstuffs, periods of over-indulgence alternate with periods of starvation. The groups they examined were sedentary, unlike the G!ãg!ai [JENKINS, BOTHA and NURSE, publication pending], and consequently it would be unwise to extrapolate all their findings to that people. Nevertheless, BRONTË-STEWART *et al.* [1960] do emphasize that clinical stigmata of chronic protein malnutrition or of avitaminosis are very infrequent. An interesting observation was that a pulp made from nuts and beans was used as a post-weaning foodstuff for infants, and that as a result the severe post-weaning protein deficiency found in many African peoples did not occur. On the other hand, they did find the elderly to be undernourished.

The !Kung of the Dobe area of Botswana have been the subjects of nutritional studies by TRUSWELL *et al.* [1969] and TRUSWELL and HANSEN [1975]. This group is substantially included in the serogenetic sample. The San appeared to these workers to be moderately undernourished as judged by weight/height ratio and skinfold thicknesses. In their opinion, chronic or seasonal calorie insufficiency may be a major reason why the San do not reach the same adult stature as most other people. Evidence for a secular increase in San stature has been provided by TOBIAS [1962]. He relates it to improvement in the diet of those working on farms. If any seasonally recurrent shortage of food is indeed a major cause of the short stature of the San, it would nevertheless be difficult to explain the greater stature of Negroes in those areas of Africa which are subject to chronic or regular periodical famine, particularly as such famine tends to be very severe by San standards. The nomadic or cyclically migratory San, though spare in build, appear to be remarkably healthy, and show no clinical signs of deprivation of nutriment. Their haematological state, in which inadequacy of nutrition might be expected to be reflected, is entirely good [METZ *et al.*, 1971]. On the other hand, that of the settled ǂhuã:, living principally on a diet similar to that of their Negro peasant patrons and only occasionally hunting and gathering, is no better than that of Southern African Negroes, in whom it is not ideal [JENKINS *et al.*, in preparation]. It seems quite possible that stature may be related to gross caloric intake rather than to dietary balance; this could account for the secular increase and the taller Negroes, and still leave the short nomadic San in possession of a diet superior to that of their settled brothers. TRUSWELL and HANSEN [1975] come to much the same conclusion, and the data of LEE [1969] support it.

The work of TANAKA [1969, 1975] and SILBERBAUER [1965] shows that there can be a dramatic fall in nutritional status among the G/wi and G//ana towards the middle of summer in years when the rains are late, but that in general the diet is various, protein-rich and at least adequate if not abundant. WEHMEYER *et al.* [1969] have provided an account of the nutrient value of the vegetable foods of the !Kung, and found them to be high; they conclude that a combination of only a particular three could supply a sufficient diet.

There is abundant information on the diet, though little on the nutritional status, of hunter-gatherer groups in Angola. ESTERMANN [1956] describes the Kwisi as hunting all animals except the lion and the buffalo. He states that the women sometimes cultivate small maize gardens with stone implements. As with the Cimba, the men gather honey and the women fruits. The Kwadi keep a few milch cattle, consume milk, and, though they do not hunt much, fish in the lagoons. The women have gardens, apparently more extensive and more varied in crops than those of the Kwisi, but still limited. Their partiality for Portuguese wine is commented on by ALMEIDA [1965], who states that they prefer the red to the white.

ALMEIDA mentions the robustness of the Kwengo of Angola, who also possess a few cattle and cultivate to a limited extent, though they depend mainly on hunting and gathering for food. These Kwengo live in encampments, and may be described as semi-sedentary. Though he criticizes the alimentary improvidence of the !Kung, GUERREIRO [1968] admits that actual death from hunger is extremely rare. He describes them as a people undernourished during the greater part of the year, but states that victuals indispensable to a balanced diet are never lacking. He differs from most other writers in claiming that their vegetable foods are of low nutritional value, but since he mentions the highly nutritive *mangeti* nut and a number of root vegetables, his lack of specific knowledge of the field of nutrition may have misled him. It certainly has when he adduces the gracefulness and torpor of the San as evidences of their being undernourished.

Neither RIBAS [n.d.] nor REDINHA [1974], dealing with dietary and hunting practices in Angola, provides any relevant information.

Growth and Physique

Studies of the physique of the San, Khoi and Cimba are included among those classical physical anthropological investigations to which reference has been made, and which have been summarized, earlier. The results of the anthropometry carried out on the Dama by KNUSSMANN are not available to us in detail, but he includes in his 1969 account of them a summary of his 'somatological impressions and findings'. He states that they have 'a certain somatological distinctiveness' among the Negroid peoples of South West Africa, and are characterized by relatively long trunks, small faces, steep foreheads, moderate stature, a tendency to mesocephaly and a dark skin. Though these features in themselves may not convey any clear idea of their distinctiveness, it is certainly true that the Dama 'look' unlike the other South West African Negroes. ALMEIDA [1965] comments on the Negroid physique of the Kwengo, and GUERREIRO [1968] has added nothing new to our knowledge of the San physique.

TRUSWELL and HANSEN [1975] have compared the heights and weights of !Kung children with those in the Harvard growth curves. For the first year of life, 50–60% were within the normal range, but after the end of the first year most children dropped below the third percentile in weight and height, a tendency aggravated between the ages of 6 and 12 years. In adolescence, weight and height remained low and comparable with adult values. It therefore appears that though San infants compare favourably with Caucasoid ones, after weaning there is a retardation of growth persisting into adult life. TRUSWELL and HANSEN suggest that there is an energy deficit throughout the growing period and that this could account for the adult stature.

Unusual Metabolic Features of the San

The long period of differentiation of the San from other races has led a number of workers to look for unusual features in their metabolic processes. In view of their widespread distribution until comparatively recently, the San habitus cannot represent a specific adaptation to a desert environment, as TOBIAS [1957] has pointed out, and these metabolic oddities are likely to have arisen, like the anatomical peculiarities, in the main through drift. The temptation to find adaptive explanations is, however, constantly present and frequently indulged.

Carbohydrate Metabolism

The capacity of the Dobe !Kung to dispose of an oral glucose load, and their hormonal response to it, have been studied by JOFFE *et al.* [1971]. They found that 15 adult !Kung showed relative glucose intolerance and significantly impaired insulin secretion, but no difference in growth hormone response, when compared with 10 non-obese Caucasoid controls. JENKINS *et al.* [1974] found lower fasting blood sugars but a similar prolonged rise following glucose ingestion by six Tsumkwe !Kung subjects. A rise similarly prolonged, though not as pronounced, was found in 5 of 11 !Xõ subjects. A twelfth was frankly diabetic [JENKINS *et al.*, in preparation]. These series can all be criticized on the grounds of possible protracted carbohydrate deprivation in the subjects prior to the tests, which would lead to a longer than normal elevation of blood glucose. It is nevertheless possible that the unusual glucose-tolerance curves of the San may indicate that increased consumption of sugar could induce clinical diabetes mellitus in them. It is perhaps not irrelevant that the elderly !Xõ woman so afflicted does have easy access to a trading store which sells sugar.

Serum Lipids

The serum lipids of the San have been found to be very low. TOBIAS [1966] first reported a mean concentration of 121 mg cholesterol per 100 ml, and subsequent studies have supplied similar or even lower values. The high linoleic acid content of the widely consumed *mangeti* nut may be responsible for this. The San are characterized also by low levels of serum triglycerides and phospholipids. The populations so far investigated, an unspecified hunting party from southern Botswana, almost certainly !Xõ [MILLER *et al.*, 1968], the Nharo and //au//en of Ghanzi district in western Botswana [BERSOHN and TOBIAS, unpublished, quoted in TOBIAS, 1966] and the !Kung of the Dobe area in north-western Botswana [TRUSWELL and HANSEN, 1968a, 1975; TRUSWELL and MANN, 1972] all resembled one another in this respect, though methodological differences make the series of MILLER *et al.* not strictly comparable with the rest. BERSOHN and TOBIAS found that San settled and working on farms, and thus in receipt of food similar to that eaten by Negroes, had cholesterol levels higher than those of the nomads. This helps to confirm the suggestion that dietary rather than inherited tendencies are responsible. Even the fat of the game animals consumed by the San is less saturated and contains higher proportions of polyunsaturated fatty acids than that of domesticated meat animals.

Blood Pressure

The number and complexity of the factors affecting the arterial blood pressure are such that no precise conclusions can be reached about the causes of its distribution in a population. There do tend, nonetheless, to be significant overall differences between the means of various peoples. The systolic and diastolic blood pressures in the San of south-western Botswana, presumably !Xõ or Nharo or related groups, were found by KAMINER and LUTZ [1960] to be lower than in Caucasoids, Negroes, Australian Aborigines and Eskimos, and comparable with those in the Chinese. Blood pressures in semi-settled San (prisoners and farm labourers) were higher than those in nomads and there was apparently no increase with ageing. TRUSWELL *et al.* [1972] reported that in the Dobe !Kung ageing was actually associated with a decrease in the blood pressures of the men, while in the women the systolic pressure showed a small rise and the diastolic a slight fall after the menopause. They suggest that a low salt intake and lack of obesity, combined with relative freedom from mental stress, might be responsible. These findings and opinions are reaffirmed by TRUSWELL and HANSEN [1975]. They found that 6 of their !Kung subjects had urinary sodium and chloride levels only one sixth to one fifth those of Caucasoid controls. They estimated the mean daily intake of sodium chloride as about 2 g.

Serum Proteins

It might be expected that the high protein diet of the San would protect them against any of the consequences of protein deprivation, and indeed the mean total serum protein concentrations which have been reported have been high normal [BERSOHN and TOBIAS, unpublished, quoted in TOBIAS, 1966; BRONTË-STEWART *et al.*, 1960; TRUSWELL and HANSEN, 1975]. The albumin/globulin ratio tends nevertheless to be low, as do mean albumin levels. The details are shown in table XXV; it will be seen that this phenomenon is due, at least in part, to an increase in the levels of γ-globulin. It has been suggested [JOFFE, personal commun., 1974] that the low albumin levels may be responsible, at least in part, for the abnormal glucose tolerance curves.

Exogenous Diseases

The precise range of exogenous causes of disease to which the hunter-gatherers of Southern Africa are exposed has not yet been determined. According to the medical staff at Tsumkwe, pulmonary tuberculosis is very prevalent among the !Kung there, and it is said to be spreading even in such remote Central Botswana groups as the G/wi and G//ana [TANAKA, personal commun.] and in the !Xõ of the south [HEINZ, 1962]. TRUSWELL and HANSEN *able XXV.* Serum proteins in San populations

opulation	n	Total protein, g%	Albumin, g%	Globulin, g% total	α_1	α_2	β	γ	Reference
1ainly Central, Ghanzi area									
Nomadic	27	8.02	2.80	5.22	0.47	0.97	1.19	2.59	BERSOHN and TOBIAS, unpublished, quoted in TOBIAS [1966]
Farm	63	7.91	3.19	4.72	0.45	0.94	1.17	2.16	as above
Kung of Kavango	94	8.24	3.46	4.78	0.39	0.75	0.96	2.68	BRONTË-STEWART *et al.* [1960]
Kung of Tsumkwe	45	7.37	3.73	3.64		1.54		2.10	TRUSWELL and HANSEN [1975]

[1975] confirm its presence among the !Kung at Dobe, and BRONTË-STEWART *et al.* [1960] found evidence of its occurrence among the !Kung of the Kavango.

Extravenereal syphilis is the most commonly encountered of the other microbial diseases. This condition has long been known to have a high prevalence in Botswana, particularly among the Kgalagadi [MURRAY *et al.*, 1952; MURRAY, 1957]; it has more recently been reported at high frequencies among the G/wi and G//ana [NURSE *et al.*, 1973]. There is evidence, not yet fully analyzed, which suggests that venereal syphilis is present in the more settled groups; HEINZ [1962] has suggested that this represents spread from Negroes, but the channel of infection with *T. pallidum* is so environmentally regulated [HUDSON, 1958] that it may have resulted simply from sedentarization.

Rabies is endemic in the small rodents of Southern Africa, but no case of human rabies in hunter-gatherers has been reported. Plague spreads periodically among rodents from a focus in Oŵambo, where it is endemic, and an investigation of plague antibodies in all the neighbouring populations has been commenced.

Some epidemic diseases can be devastating, due to the absence of previous exposure. There are no accounts of the responses to the minor exanthemata, though the severity assumed by these diseases in other African groups suggests that they probably constitute a danger, particularly to children. A smallpox epidemic ravaged the inhabitants of the Kalahari in 1950/51, with reportedly high mortality among the San [SILBERBAUER, 1965]. Poliomyelitis antibodies have been found in a large sample of !Xõ from the Lone Tree area [JENKINS *et al.*, 1968]. Influenza spreads regularly from the settlements, and though the effects are rapid and severe it does not often appear to be fatal [HEINZ, 1962]. KOKERNOT *et al.* [1965] have carried out a survey of the prevalence of antibodies against arthropod-borne viruses; unfortunately, the populations from which the sera were drawn are not specified, but from the localities at which these were taken they might be expected to include hunter-gatherers. They found evidence of the presence of quite a wide variety of viruses, with Sindbis in group A and West Nile in group B the commonest. These two, and Wesselsbron in group B, appeared to be the only ones occurring in the very dry environments; Semliki and Chikungunya of group A, and H. 336 and Spondweni in group B, as well as Bunyamwera and Germiston in the Bunyamwera group, were found in addition in the Okavango Basin and the Caprivi Strip. Another viral disease which has been found to attain quite a high prevalence among hunter-gatherers, type B hepatitis, is treated at greater length below. It furnishes an informative model of the modes of spread of infectious disease in these populations.

Malaria is of course endemic in the areas of the Kavango river and delta. It is surprisingly common in the Kalahari as a whole; when the rains come, the shallow warm pans form an eminently suitable breeding-ground for mosquitos. BRONTË-STEWART *et al.* [1960] record that the prevalence of splenomegaly diminishes among the Northern !Kung as distance from the river increases. The presence of both *P. falciparum* and *P. vivax* malaria at Dobe is recorded by TRUSWELL and HANSEN [1975]. With local variations, conditions similar to those at Dobe obtain for all the other Kalahari populations. Malaria seems not to occur, or at least not to be common, on the Brandberg edge of the Namib among the Dama, and nothing is known for certain about its incidence in the Cimba. No certain case of trypanosomiasis has been diagnosed, to our knowledge, in a hunter-gatherer; but in late 1972, one of us confirmed the presence of *T. rhodesiense* in the blood of a Caucasoid missionary living in the Kavango Valley and in touch with both Kwengo and G!ãg!ai. The vector, the tsetse fly *Glossina morsitans*, is common in the area, and the disease almost certainly occurs. The missionary was flown to Cape Town, and recovered. Other patients are probably not so fortunate.

Serological evidence of toxoplasmosis has been found in several of these populations: 12.1% of the G/wi and G//ana gave positive reactions, 7.3% of the ‡huã:, who share much the same ecosystem, 6.2% of the !Kung of Tsumkwe and 9.1% of the Dobe !Kung. Among the Dama, the figure was the significantly higher one ($\chi^2_{[1]} = 25.6$, $p<0.001$) of 27.3% [MASON *et al.*, publication pending]. All of these populations except the Dama hunt and eat wild felids, but none of them keeps domestic cats. It is suggested by MASON *et al.* that the comparatively sedentary life of the Dama would attract wild felids and rodents to the middens, and that oocysts would consequently tend to accumulate in the vicinity of the settlements. The !Kung, ǂhuã: and !Xõ are marginally more sedentary than the G/wi and G//ana, whose higher figure may be due to higher consumption of wild felids.

The most conspicuous of all the exogenous diseases is *witkop,* white head, or favus. It is found particularly in the San, and it had long been assumed by casual workers in the field that it was a syphiloderm. The frequency with which it was found in association with seropositivity for syphilis seemed to confirm this. A careful epidemiological study by MURRAY *et al.* [1967] demonstrated, however, that it was primarily infection with *Trichophyton schoenleinii,* a fungus. It is extremely common, particularly in children; it tends to regress at puberty, leaving, in many cases, bald patches.

Purulent conjunctivitis is frequently seen in hunter-gatherers, and is probably exacerbated by smoke and the exsiccation of the conjunctiva due to sitting close to fires. BRONTË-STEWART *et al.* [1960] confirmed the presence of trachoma in the northern !Kung, and it is almost certainly present in many other groups. We have observed it in the G/wi and in the Denasena. Periodontal infection is common, but dental caries is rare; dental erosion due to a constant coarse diet does, however, erode the crowns of the teeth and expose the dentine [VAN REENEN, 1966]. The only helminth hitherto identified in these populations is the hookworm *Necator americanus,* a somewhat surprising introduction [METZ *et al.,* 1971]. In the rest of Africa the prevailing hookworm is *Ancylostoma duodenale.* BRONTË-STEWART *et al.* [1960] mention one case of haematuria probably due to schistosomiasis, but bilharzia is relatively uncommon in the Kalahari, even in settled Negro populations [GELDENHUYS *et al.,* 1967].

TRUSWELL and HANSEN [1975] record that tonsillitis, rheumatic fever and mitral valve disease are relatively common, and the rheumatic aetiology of such cardiac disease as does occur in the San tends to be confirmed by the findings of KENNELLY *et al.* [1972].

Trauma must account for a large proportion of the ill health among hunter-gatherers. Burns, especially of children, result from crowding and jostling around the fire in winter. Thorns, and particularly the hard burnt stalks of *Grewia* bushes, are responsible for the very common puncture wounds and gashes of the feet. The conditions needed to keep the band coherent make hunter-gatherers unusually peaceable and accommodating, but fights do occur; though HEINZ [1962, 1967], an observer more qualified than most, records no old injuries due to these. Fights with wild animals, particularly leopard and lion, often leave the survivors with bizarre deformities. TRUSWELL and HANSEN [1975] mention a San man who performed a below-knee amputation on himself after being injured with a poisoned arrow. He survived.

We have seen a large breast tumour with axillary lymph node enlargement in a 50-year-old woman near Xangwa, and presume that it was a carcinoma. TANAKA and JENKINS [personal observation, 1974] encountered a similar case at ǂKade, and the woman died within two weeks.

The Epidemiology of Hepatitis B in Hunter-Gatherers

Australia antigen is of peculiar interest in the study of hunter-gatherer populations, since it was in the serum of a member of one such, an Australian aborigine, that it was first detected [BLUMBERG, 1964]. It also furnishes a particularly good example of the ease with which a non-genetic trait may appear to be Mendelianly inherited [BLUMBERG *et al.,* 1965]. Among the first sera tested were some from a large Samaritan kinship, and these together with two instances of family clustering found in sera from the Marshall Islands suggested that the antigen was inherited as a simple autosomal recessive trait. A subsequent study in the Philippines provided strong supportive evidence for this hypothesis [BLUMBERG *et al.,* 1966]. This was later, however, modified into one of recessive inheritance of susceptibility to infection by the antigen [BLUMBERG *et al.,* 1969]. The antigen has now been recognized as a transmissible infective agent probably responsible for viral hepatitis, serum hepatitis or type B [PRINCE, 1968] and consequently as a blood transfusion hazard [GOCKE, 1970].

Serum or type B hepatitis may be transmitted by any procedure in which the infective agent can enter the body through a skin or mucosal puncture. It also appears probable that it may be transmitted by ingestion [ZUCKERMAN, 1972]. In Western communities, it is uncommon in children except in institutions, while in apparently healthy populations in the underdeveloped countries it may be present in 10–20% of the population. Where it is not associated with transfusion or other forms of venepuncture, it has a long incubation period, 60–180 days or even longer.

Among the hunter-gatherer groups of Southern Africa, an unusually high prevalence of hepatitis B antigen has been found in the G/wi and G//ana [NURSE *et al.,* 1973]. Their figure is 14%, as compared with 9% of Botswana Negroes, 10.3% of the !Kung of Botswana, 10% of the Kwengo and only 2.7% of the G!ãg!ai [BERSOHN *et al.,* 1974]. The combined figure for the G/wi and G//ana in fact masks a surprising difference between them: the prevalence is 18% in the G/wi and only 6% in the G//ana, and the difference generates $\chi^2_{[1]}$ of 5.01, $p<0.05$. We report here the results of two separate surveys of the Tsumkwe !Kung, in June 1971 and May 1974, which gave prevalences of 9.2 and 4.2%, respectively; but sample sizes were far from identical, and $\chi^2_{[1]}$ was only 1.18. The !Xõ have the highest prevalence yet to be reported in a Southern African population, 26%, but the sample consisted of only 46 individuals. The ‡huã: prevalence is 11.4%, and that of the Dama 7%.

In Southern African hunter-gatherer populations, the maintenance of hygiene depends largely on the degree of isolation from other peoples, low population density, frequent shifts of living sites and to some extent solar irradiation. Even when the living sites are fairly static, at times of plenty, the freely deposited and unburied faeces are rapidly disposed of by the numerous dung beetles *(Scarabaeus spp.)* which either bury or consume them. Little trouble is taken to keep food clean, but then food is usually consumed fresh. Despite their reputation for being dirty people, most San wash whenever water is available; in the absence of water, before meals, they will wash their hands in urine [SILBERBAUER, 1965]. There is little doubt that faecal contamination of foodstuffs can take place, either through handling or carriage by flies *(Musca spp.)*, and this is one probable mode of spread for the hepatitis B antigen once it has become established in a member of a band. Another is the likelihood that in a crowded camp more than one person may be punctured or scratched by the same thorn or twig. This route of infection has been postulated as a reason for the occurrence of epidemics of hepatitis among Swedish cross-country runners [GABINUS and JONSSON, 1962] and it would appear even more relevant under hunter-gatherer conditions in Southern Africa.

Evidence that the occurrence of type B hepatitis among the Kalahari San is epidemic has been provided by sub-typing of the Australia antigen found in the G/wi and the G//ana [LE BOUVIER *et al.*, in preparation]. Sub-typing was carried out on 17 persons above and 5 below 10 years old among the G/wi, and 3 over 10 years old among the G//ana. All of those over 10 years old had the d sub-type of the antigen, and all of those below the y sub-type. The eldest individual with the y sub-type was a G/wi boy of about 9 years; the youngest with d a G//ana girl of about 12. The approximate age-range of the d-positive G/wi was 22–55 years, and the other two G//ana were about 22 and 28 years old. Though it would be impossible to date the introduction of the d strain into the population without further information, it would appear to have occurred more than 10 years prior to 1972, the year in which the specimens were taken, and it is highly probable that the y strain would have been introduced in about 1962.

It has fortunately been possible to obtain some contributory evidence about the latter phenomenon. In 1963, a certain well-known writer and anthropologist, referred to elsewhere in these pages, suffered an attack of 'infectious hepatitis' while working among the G/wi. Ten years later he kindly supplied us with a specimen of his serum which, however, proved not to contain Australia antigen. It is nevertheless likely that he could have been the agent of entry of the new strain into the population, particularly as it was found exclusively among the G/wi and not in the G//ana. It is to be presumed that the previous exposure of the older people to the d type antigen would have protected them against the new strain, which would have continued to be passed on among the children after the anthropologist had left.

It is improbable that he could have been the only person to introduce the y strain into the Kalahari. Of the 23 !Xõ with antibodies against Australia antigen, 3 had antibodies against y, as did one of the 10 ‡huã:. The age distribution was not revealing in these populations, which have much more contact with Kgalagadi than the G/wi and G//ana have. Unfortunately, there are no data on either antigen or antibody among the Kgalagadi, whose migrations, when they migrate, tend to bring them into fairly frequent contact with settled Negroes. The predominance of the y strain among the Kavango Negroes, who have fairly close contact with the !Kung of South West Africa, could account for the finding of 8 of the latter with antibodies against y as against 35 with antibodies against d only out of the combined sample of 220.

The most usual routes of introduction of the antigen would seem to be those by which most 'foreign' infective agents enter these populations. Purely migrant groups have cyclical contacts with related settled and semi-settled groups, with one another, and with hunters and others who pay brief visits to their areas. They are also beginning to make increasing use of trading stores. Some men from any of these kinds of groups may extend their migrations to include periods of employment well away from their own areas, even on the industrial and crowded Witwatersrand. Anyone with no previous resistance to the infections latent in concentrations of population may return to his own people with a variety of micro-organisms which he will distribute among those with whom he comes in contact. It seems that the human vector is probably the most dangerous agent of the spread of infectious diseases among hunter-gatherers.

Inherited Diseases

There are few published accounts of inherited disease in Southern African hunter-gatherers, and what there are relate entirely to the San. BEIGHTON [1972] described pituitary dwarfism in a single 'Mokoko' (!Xõ) man, with normal parents and siblings, but was unable to say whether it was genetic in aetiology. In 1952, TOBIAS [personal commun., 1974] had seen the same case and another on an adjoining farm near Ghanzi. The cases differed, however, in genital development and secondary sexual characteristics, and it does not appear likely that they represented two manifestations of the same condition.

Another unpublished 1952 observation by TOBIAS was that of an albino San, the only one so far recorded. Despite the claim by the informants of SILBERBAUER [1956] that twinning does not occur among the San, Prof. TOBIAS has kindly furnished us with a photograph of a pair of San twins taken during the same expedition. Another photograph, of an Angola !Kung mother with twins, may be found in GUERREIRO [1968].

We have carried out a family study on a case of Treacher-Collins syndrome among the Tsumkwe !Kung, and have observed a 10-year-old boy with microcephaly, polydactyly and mental retardation among the !Kung of Dobe. Supernumerary nipples, and rudimentary non-functional breasts along the milk line, are sometimes observed in the San.

Considering the sizes of the San populations, it is hardly surprising that there is so restricted a range of inherited pathological conditions on record. We have been given anecdotal assurances that an obviously defective infant born away from places accessible to government agencies would probably be killed soon after birth. Though such a practice would not have any marked effect on the frequency in the population of the gene for a recessively inherited condition of large effect, it would naturally mask the presence of such genes from observers. It is nonetheless surprising that Down's syndrome has not been reported even among the settled farm San or those at Tsumkwe or Dobe.

We have not been able to find any account of inherited disease among other Southern African hunter-gatherer populations.

Chapter 6. Population Structure among the Southern African Hunter-Gatherers

The diversity of structure among the hunting and gathering populations of Southern Africa is to a great extent attributable to the rather broad boundaries we have set to that form of culture in this monograph. We have drawn no firm distinction between hunting and gathering and a sedentary life, principally because so many settled or semi-settled populations would be unable to survive, or at least to flourish, solely on the products of their husbandry or the rewards of their labour. Even the most extreme groups, those which hunt and gather all their food and raiment, do enter into some barter arrangements with other populations, and thereby obtain such commodities as tobacco and, increasingly, metal (and plastic) implements, sugar and coloured beads. We can therefore divide these populations into two main categories, those who are purely migrant, such as the G/wi and G//ana of the central Kalahari, a majority of the Hei//om and Kwengo, some Dama groups around the Brandberg, the !Xõ in the south and certain of the Zhu/oasi (!Kung) of northern Botswana, southern Angola and the north-east of South West Africa, and the rest, all of whom live a settled life either permanently or for part of the year.

Migrant Hunter-Gatherers

Migration among hunter-gatherers is regulated by the presence of concentrations of game and the availability of food plants, and to some extent by the presence of water. The last-named consideration is more important to some groups than to others: whereas the !Kung migrants move from waterhole to waterhole [Lee, 1965], the G/wi [Silberbauer, 1965] and the G//ana [Tanaka, 1969, 1975] depend to a greater extent on plants, particularly the *tsamma* melon, and perhaps on the rumen of their prey, for water. Availability of resources limits social organization to the level of the band, which generally consists of around 50 individuals. That this size of band necessarily applies to virtually all hunter-gatherer populations has been pointed out by WILMSEN [1973]. Membership of a band is permanent, but an individual, or a family, can belong to more than one band and follow an idiosyncratic migration pattern, changing bands where the routes coincide. Membership of a San band entails rights but not obligations [MARSHALL, 1960]; failure to conform to an acceptable pattern can, however, lead to ostracism and voluntary abnegation of association by the person or group ostracized [TANAKA, personal commun.; SILBERBAUER, 1965, personal commun.; see above]. Joining a new band involves establishing inherited membership rights or being accepted by the bands as a marriage partner for one of its members, or simply agreement with the people of the band as a whole.

When a band grows to an unwieldy or economically unviable size, there is either gradual erosion of its membership or fission of a whole segment which moves off to find other territory. The break is never sudden: exploration parties set out to examine alternative territories, or individuals or families make slow contact with smaller bands which they wish to join, and eventually the change has taken place, the pressures are relieved, and the band has returned to a more suitable size. In the process there has been either the formation of a new band, or marked change in and expansion of the membership of such bands as happen to be close at the time, or both. Movement of population to new territory is always entailed; there would be no economic justification for simple division of rights over the existing territory. On the other hand catastrophes, such as the smallpox epidemic of 1950–51, can decimate the population to the extent that survivors of several bands amalgamate into one, and thereby amass a large enough territory to provide open lands when growth of numbers once more leads to fission. SILBERBAUER [1965] estimates that fission generally takes place once every two or three generations, and that in the absence of abnormal constraints the net annual increase in population is consequently of the order of 2.5%.

Marriage is a matter of concern to the band even more than it is to the individuals, and marriages have to be consented to by the whole community. Matings between members of the band are preferred to exogamy, though small numbers often mean that marriageable age is reached when no partner of the opposite sex is available, and mates may then be sought from outside. It is usual for the husband to join the wife's band for a probationary period, during which the marriage can be dissolved simply by the husband's departure. After the birth of the first child the couple may, and often does, remove to the husband's tribe. Polygamy is practised to a greater or lesser extent in various groups. Divorce is not common among the G/wi, but the !Kung frequently speak of having had several successive wives or husbands.

Since the rights of a woman are equal to those of a man, she is as entitled as he is to dissolve the marriage. Another relationship of genetic importance is the hunting bond between men. Men usually hunt in pairs; very young men change their hunting partners frequently, but as they mature a permanent bond between pairs of men develops. This results in classificatory siblinghood among their offspring; marriage to the child of a father's hunting partner is regarded as incestuous, and avoided, but the theoretical kinship endures for only a single generation. Another consequence is that mature married men do not change bands alone, but always together with their families and the families of their hunting partners.

The foregoing applies in the main to all the San groups, to the Hei//om and to the Kwengo. It appears not to apply to the Dama, who according to VEDDER [1923] had as their principal social unit the extended family, which functioned as a band. As a result band exogamy was, and in such small migrant Dama groups as survive probably still is, the rule. The Dama profess Christianity and avoid overt polygamy. Little appears to be known of their present social structure, and it is impossible to do more than speculate about the forces which now regulate gene flow in them. DORNAN [1922] states that the Denasena have totemic and isonymic exogamy, and the persistence of this has lately been confirmed [CHASKO, personal commun.]. In fact it appears that the Denasena are beginning to accommodate themselves to Tswana *mores,* and that their population structure is in the process of being altered by mass sedentarization.

Settled Hunter-Gatherers

It is possible to recognize three main types of settled hunter-gatherers:

1) Farmers whose produce is insufficient to maintain them throughout the year. The Khoi of Sesfontein and the Kuiseb Valley, the Kwisi, the Kwadi, most of the Denasena and many of the Dama would be included in this class.

2) Labourers working for part of the year on farms and for the rest periodically migrant. Among these we would include such San groups as the ǂhuã:, who live as clients of the Kgalagadi, the !Kung of Ngami and the G!aokx'ate of Gobabis who have similar relationships with Herero, those !Kung in Grootfontein and Tsumeb districts and the G!aokx'ate of Gobabis district in South West Africa, and many of the Nharo, //au//en and G//ana of Ghanzi district in Botswana, who work on the farms of Caucasoids,

and the Dama seasonal workers in many parts of South West Africa. Some Kgalagadi live in a semi-permanent clientage relationship with settled Tswana.

3) Persons living in permanent settlements in the immediate or accessible vicinity of which sufficient food may be hunted and gathered throughout the year, and consequently practising neither regular migration nor husbandry. The !Kung of Dobe, /du/da, /ai/ai and Tsumkwe would fall into this class, at least in part, though numbers of them either migrate seasonally or make long forays in search of particular foods. LEE [1965] has pointed out that migration is not necessarily due to shortage of food and that particularly in the Dobe area there is an abundance of food throughout the year; the incentive can be simply a wish to visit other bands or a desire for a different range of foodstuffs.

It is plain that the factors determining the genetic structures of these various types of population must differ considerably. The settled farmers of the kind inhabiting the Kuiseb Valley, for instance, might be expected to represent virtual isolates, with intensive drift compounded by small population size and enforced endogamy; while the small size of the migrant bands will provoke the contrary trend, with comparatively frequent exogamy and consequent gene exchange with other bands which are for part of the year, or in some years, geographically remote. HARPENDING and JENKINS [1973] emphasize the resulting uniformity among the San, who display less evidence of band isolation than do, for instance, the settled Coloured (mixed) communities of the northern Cape Province.

HARPENDING and JENKINS [1974] and HARPENDING [1975] have dealt with genetic variation in Zhu/oasi (!Kung) populations, which include true migrants and the two latter types of settled and semi-settled peoples. They found that when the amount of genetic variation was compared with that predicted by known migration and mating practices, a close accord existed between the observed and the expected data, and that irrespective of the migration pattern the genetic distances generated provided a good reflection of the geographic distances. It appeared from their conclusions that all types of Southern African hunter-gatherers, with the probable exception of the farmers who practise hunting and gathering only for part of the year and in the immediate neighbourhood of their settlements, would be subject to the same conditions of gene exchange and that these would relate directly to geographical distance. The range of genetic markers, and the number of populations examined, have increased, however, since their study was carried out, and several factors which tend to modify their conclusions seem to emerge from more recent studies.

Gene exchange does transcend linguistic barriers among the San of the Kalahari, and the accompanying tables suggest that the putatively Khoi Hei//om are subject to the same forces as the San and are steadily becoming more like them. Such a trend would appear to operate to an equal extent in the Negro hunter-gatherers, the Dama, Kgalagadi, Cimba, Kwisi, Kwadi, Denasena and Kwengo. The Kwengo have gene frequencies almost identical with those of their Mbukushu neighbours, from whom they are culturally and linguistically quite distinct [Nurse and Jenkins, in preparation]. Little is known of the genetic structure of the Kwisi and Kwadi, but their contacts with Negro groups appear to be more considerable than with the culturally similar San, while the Dama show little evidence of having received a Khoisan genetic contribution [Nurse *et al.*, 1976]. The Cimba have little or no contact with the Khoisan, and the sample drawn was too small for proper analysis. The Kgalagadi hold themselves to be socially superior to the San, with whom their matings are informal. Each of these groups, with the exception of the Kgalagadi and the Kwengo, is separated by non-intersection of migration paths from the San hunter-gatherers (though there is admittedly some contact between these and settled Dama in the Grootfontein and Tsumeb districts of South West Africa). Each is, in fact, culturally isolated, and gene exchange would appear to take place mainly with genetically similar and geographically close populations practising full-time husbandry.

This process may well constitute a model for the future population structure of the San. As more and more of them adopt a sedentary life permanently, relationship among the various groups is likely to become more restricted. As the Cimba, who may be migrant Himba, have their principal contacts with the Himba, as the Denasena and Kgalagadi find it progressively easier to ally and identify themselves with the Tswana, as the Kwengo, who are almost certainly socially degraded Mbukushu, come into closer touch with the Mbukushu than with anyone else, and as the hunting and gathering Dama merge almost imperceptibly into the settled Dama, so may it be anticipated that the San and Hei//om of the farms will maintain close links with the groups from which they spring which, in turn, will restrict migration in order to preserve socially and economically advantageous contact with their kin; the San, from being virtually a single people, will drift into fragments as distinct as now are the Khoi of the Kuiseb, of Sesfontein and of Keetmanshoop. The genetic distances as they are now will change, but until the patterns of gene flow into and from other peoples, and the degree of drift which will operate, are known, it is impossible to suggest how.

Genetic Distance

Among the principal considerations to be evaluated in the interpretation of any measure of genetic distance are the amount and quality of the non-genetic information available about the populations being compared. If we know from historically reliable sources that two populations descend without further admixture from a single parent population, then any measure of their overall differences is likely to be a combined measure of founder effect, of random loss of genes, and probably of selective pressures. Such straightforward conditions hold, however, for very few of the populations that are likely to come up for comparison in circumscribed regions, though they would seem to apply in the cases of comparisons between geographically remote populations, or the major races.

The Southern African hunter-gatherers can, indeed, be apportioned between the Khoisan and Negro races, but the quantity of gene exchange, even, in some cases, the very small quantity, that has taken place between them, both adds an element of perturbation to many of the distance estimations and induces caution in their interpretation. It is impossible at the present time to hypothesize with any assurance about the genetic structures of the unmixed ancestral Khoisan or Negro populations. One can be reasonably sure that certain alleles, such as A^{bantu} and acid phosphatase P^{r}, are characteristically Khoisan, and that peptidase Pep^{A2} and $Gm^{1,5,6}$ are Negro, but there remain uncertainties about, for instance, the part played by drift, or even selection, in the attainment of the present frequencies of the Henshaw antigen and PGM_2^2. It would therefore be hazardous to consider estimating exact proportions of admixture.

A number of measures of genetic distance have been proposed, and all of them have their advantages and disadvantages. These are discussed by CAVALLI-SFORZA and BODMER [1971], by GOWER [1972], by SANGHVI and BALAKRISHNAN [1972] and by JACQUARD [1974]. Largely on the advice of BODMER [personal commun., 1975], but also because it is adaptable to our somewhat limited computation facilities and because it appears to minimize the effects of sample size, we have chosen to compare certain of the populations discussed by the method of EDWARDS and CAVALLI-SFORZA [1972].

This method involves at each locus the arc-cosine transformation of the gene frequencies and the consequent situation of population points on the surface of a hypersphere. The conversion to Euclidean space is brought about by the stereographic projection of the population space on to a tangent plane equally inclined to all the original Cartesian axes. In this space, the distance at a locus between two populations with gene frequencies p_i and p_i' is given by E where:

$$E^2 = \frac{8\,(1-\Sigma\sqrt{p_i p_i'})}{(1+\Sigma\sqrt{p_i/k})\;(1+\Sigma\sqrt{p_i'/k})},$$

and k is the number of alleles at the locus. Combination of distances over loci can be accomplished by summing E^2 and dividing by $\Sigma\,(k\text{-}1)$ to give the generalized square distance.

It would appear at first sight as if the closest approximation to the 'true' genetic distance would involve using as many loci as possible in the comparisons; but, as is shown elsewhere [NURSE, in preparation] the loci actually examined include only those most accessible to investigation, which are not necessarily those which provide the most significant information. Where the differences at a locus are small, the information derived from that locus will tend to reduce the calculated distances. In comparisons between a single pair of populations this will not matter, but where a number of populations are being considered such loci can be a source of bias. Whether the introduction of opposing bias by using only those loci which are most informative is justifiable may be doubted; but since the selection of loci is in any case arbitrary, it seems reasonable to heighten the contrasts among the populations by a judicious choice of loci.

We have consequently only compared those populations for which we have data at a maximum number of informative loci. The loci at our disposal which proved to generate maximum information were ABO, MNSs Henshaw, rhesus, Duffy, first and second phosphoglucomutase, acid phosphatase, 6PGD, G6PD, haptoglobin and transferrin. We must emphasize that the information potential of these loci applies only within the population set chosen and with the array of alleles at each locus found within that population set. For instance, the *NsHe* allele was present in only two of the populations, but in comparison its absence from all the others had to be taken into account. This produced a slight reduction of contrast and of information content in comparisons among those populations in whom it did not occur.

The populations compared consisted of ten Khoisan groups, the !Xõ, ‡huã:, G/wi, G//ana, Nharo, //au//en, the !Kung of Tsumkwe G!ãg!ai, Hei//om and G!aokx'ate, and three groups of Negroes, the Dama, Kwengo and Denasena. For the //au//en, there were no data on acid phosphatase, and particulars about the transferrins of the Hei//om are lacking. The other eleven populations are compared on all systems in table XXVIa, and all 13

Table XXVIa. Genetic distances among 13 Southern African hunter-gatherer populations calculated from gene frequency data in eleven marker systems

	!Xõ	ǂhuã:	G/wi	G//ana	Nharo	//au//en[a]	Tsumkwe !Kung	G!ãg!ai	Hei//om[b]	Kwengo	Dama	Denasena
G!aokx'ate	0.0370	0.0332	0.0220	0.0411	0.0246	(0.0265)	0.0318	0.0331	(0.0359)	0.0732	0.0912	0.0744
!Xõ		0.0398	0.0098	0.0282	0.0204	(0.0221)	0.0235	0.0289	(0.0347)	0.0648	0.0817	0.0522
ǂhuã			0.0249	0.0277	0.0301	(0.0328)	0.0346	0.0333	(0.0346)	0.0637	0.0692	0.0621
G/wi				0.0138	0.0164	(0.0170)	0.0167	0.0289	(0.0228)	0.0474	0.0667	0.0421
G//ana					0.0272	(0.0280)	0.0342	0.0470	(0.0257)	0.0475	0.0623	0.0418
Nharo						(0.0082)	0.0097	0.0220	(0.0096)	0.0461	0.0565	0.0328
//au//en[a]							(0.0097)	(0.0224)	(0.0134)	(0.0644)	(0.0534)	(0.0372)
Tsumkwe !Kung								0.0164	(0.0164)	0.0507	0.0443	0.0323
G!ãg!ai									(0.0404)	0.0726	0.0881	0.0680
Hei//om[b]										(0.0323)	(0.0387)	(0.0240)
Kwengo											0.0346	0.0341
Dama												0.0199

[a] Excluding one system (acid phosphatase).
[b] Excluding one system (transferrin).

Table XXVIb. Genetic distances among 13 Southern African hunter-gatherer populations calculated from gene frequency data in nine marker systems

	!Xõ	ǂhuã:	G/wi	G//ana	Nharo	//au//en	Tsumkwe !Kung	G!ãg!ai	Hei//om	Kwengo	Dama	Denasena
G!aokx'ate	0.0307	0.0327	0.0197	0.0375	0.0193	0.0230	0.0225	0.0287	0.0320	0.0660	0.0730	0.0663
!Xõ		0.0405	0.0092	0.0304	0.0204	0.0229	0.0224	0.0299	0.0352	0.0698	0.0755	0.0829
ǂhuã:			0.0257	0.0288	0.0289	0.0296	0.0292	0.0329	0.0362	0.0680	0.0647	0.0596
G/wi				0.0134	0.0159	0.0170	0.0159	0.0297	0.0281	0.0480	0.0560	0.0364
G//ana					0.0247	0.0272	0.0291	0.0471	0.0237	0.0489	0.0573	0.0335
Nharo						0.0085	0.0102	0.0247	0.0099	0.0484	0.0496	0.0324
//au//en							0.0094	0.0233	0.0134	0.0654	0.0510	0.0385
Tsumkwe !Kung								0.0173	0.0174	0.0508	0.0319	0.0308
G!ãg!ai									0.0436	0.0803	0.0873	0.0729
Hei//om										0.0344	0.0355	0.0233
Kwengo											0.0349	0.0354
Dama												0.0183

populations are compared on all systems except acid phosphatase and transferrin in table XXVIb. The information content at the transferrin locus is small – it exceeds only that for PGM_2 – and failure to consider acid phosphatase is responsible for most of the differences between the two tables. This is particularly marked where the interpopulation comparisons are also comparisons between the two races.

The interracial contrasts are immediately obvious. The three Negro populations constitute a cluster representing the furthest distances from all the Khoisan populations except the G//ana and Hei//om, and this suggests that these two populations have received a larger Negro contribution than the rest of the San. This conclusions is borne out, in the case of the G//ana, by the results in individual systems where racially fairly specific alleles are segregating, but the relationships of the Hei//om are particularly puzzling. These seem, in fact, to furnish one of the most cogent excuses for our assuming that they are Khoi rather than San. Their comparative closeness to the Denasena, and the fact that they speak related languages, may indicate that their ancestors have had more contact in the past than their present geographical situations suggest. The closest populations genetically and geographically to the Hei//om are the Nharo, //au//en and Tsumkwe !Kung, who otherwise appear to form a cluster, transcending the quite distinct linguistic barriers between Northern, Central and Southern Bush, with the !Xõ and G/wi. The closest populations to the ≠huã: are the G/wi and the G//ana, and their likeness to the latter corroborates the likelihood that they, too, have received some Negro admixture. The remaining two San populations, the G!ãg!ai and G!aokx'ate, are those lying most remote from the Negro populations; they are not, however, particularly close to one another, and would seem rather to lie at the periphery of the main San cluster, but contralaterally. It appears likely that they have received less Negro genetic contribution than the other San populations, and the contrasts between them, which might be extended to the !Xõ, could be more revealing of the effects of random genetic drift among the San than the comparisons among other San populations are.

For all three of the Negro populations the affinities are in the first instance with one another; though the Hei//om, Tsumkwe !Kung and Nharo are all closer to the Denasena than the Kwengo are, the Denasena are in fact closer to the Kwengo than is any other population except the Hei//om. The comparative closeness of the Hei//om to all three Negro populations furnishes more evidence that Negro admixture has been more considerable in them than in any other San population. The affinities of the Denasena, on the other hand, reveal that they have probably received considerably more San admixture than either the Kwengo or the Dama, though in the overall comparisons they figure as unequivocally Negro.

Genetic distance calculations have consequently provided further evidence to support our contention that the Kwengo and the Denasena, hitherto regarded as 'Bushmen', are sufficiently remote from the San to be accounted members of another major race, and sufficiently close to the Dama to be considered as of the same race as they. These calculations have also helped us to show that though the San are in the main a homogeneous people, there are suggestions of genetic clines among them unrelated to linguistic differences. Scrutiny of the individual systems is helpful in delineating these clines more precisely.

Gene Flow and Frequency Clines

If in the first instance, we exclude the three Negro populations from consideration, and begin by considering the ABO system, we find that the Nharo, //au//en, G!aokx'ate and Tsumkwe and G!ãg!ai !Kung all have considerably higher frequencies of the alleles determining the stronger A antigens than the other five populations, though the Hei//om frequency is moderately high. Furthermore, the G!ãg!ai and the G!aokx'ate have frequencies of A^{bantu} greatly in excess of those in any of the other populations. The populations which lie along the western margin of the Kalahari, with the exception of the Hei//om, consequently represent a high frequency cline for A^1 and A^{int}, with the peaks of A^{bantu} at the northern and southern extremes.

A different type of cline appears from the MN system. Here low frequencies of N appear to characterize the southernmost San populations (!Xõ, G!aokx'ate, G/wi, G//ana and Nharo) with the exception of the rather easterly ǂhuã:, while the exception to the high N frequencies in the north is the Hei//om. The rhesus system appears to disclose a focus of R^2 in the most easterly San, the G//ana and ǂhuã:, falling off sharply in the neighbouring peoples and absent from the G!aokx'ate, !Xõ and G!ãg!ai, while r is confined to the western cluster and the Hei//om, though it is not found in the northernmost group, the G!ãg!ai, or the southernmost, the G!aokx'ate. Its apparent absence from so small a sample of G!ãg!ai does not mean that it is not there; in a sample of 36 the frequency of r could be 0.2 or higher without a homozygote being found. The Duffy system is not very informative here, apart from the extent to which the low Fy^a frequency in the Hei//om once more sets that group apart.

A westerly focus can be detected for the transferrin allele Tf^{D^1}, with frequencies highest in the Tsumkwe !Kung, the //au//en and the Nharo and only a little lower in the G!ãg!ai. The reduction or absence to the east and south is not consistent, as there is a moderate amount in the !Xõ. The haptoglobins show no regular pattern, though the low frequency of Hp^2 in the G!aokx'ate is puzzling. Nor is there much of interest in the G6PD and 6PGD systems. The frequency of PGM_2^2 at the second phosphoglucomutase locus seems to tend to be higher in the south, though it is lower in the G!aokx'ate than in the Nharo and was not found in the ǂhuã:. Perhaps the most striking contrast between north and south is in the frequency of P^b in the acid phosphatase system; the five southernmost populations all have much lower frequencies than the four northern populations in which it has been tested for.

Rare alleles can sometimes be more informative than their comparatively small contribution to the genetic distance might suggest [NURSE, 1974]. The haemoglobin gene $Hb\beta^{D\ Bushman}$ reaches its highest frequency in the //au//en, and it seems to have diffused from them into the !Kung to the north-east (but not due north) and the Nharo to the south and west. The !Kung of Tsumkwe and the //Hei//om are the only San with PGM_1^7 at the first phosphoglucomutase locus, while PGM_1^6 has been found only in the Tsumkwe and G!ãg!ai !Kung. The latter very probably represents gene flow from the Sesfontein Khoi, in whom it reaches the unusual frequency of 0.048. Another indication of gene flow between the Tsumkwe !Kung and the Hei//om is the finding of the peptidase $PepD^3$ allele in both of them, while coupling of the Henshaw antigen with *Ns* is found only in the Hei//om and the //au//en. The rare PGD^R allele in the 6PGD system is so characteristic of the Dama [JENKINS and NURSE, 1974] that its absence from the San is a good indication that the Negro gene flow they have received has not been from the Dama, while its presence at high frequency in the Sesfontein Topnaar but not the other Khoi suggests that gene flow from the Dama has taken place into that population.

It can be seen that though the San are in the main a uniform people there are factors which indicate biological demarcations among them. We can distinguish a group characterized by high $N, r, A^1/A^{int}$ and P^b frequencies, in the north-west; another with low frequencies of these alleles and moderate ones of PGM_2^2 in the south; and an eastern focus of R^2. Not enough is yet known about the serogenetics of the Khoi for us to be sure whether they are indeed characterized by the presence of PGM_1^6, and whether the serogenetic peculiarities of the Hei//om, such as the presence of PGM_1^7, *NsHe* and

PepD[3], may be confirmatory of our suggestion that they are Khoi rather than San. That suggestion is certainly supported by the findings in the HLA system [NURSE *et al.,* 1975].

Population Size and Population Structure

An important consideration in the structure of hunting and gathering populations is that of the effective population size. It has been shown that a strong interdependence exists between the size of a band and the quantity of available resources. For the purpose of these studies, a band must be considered a whole population. Where the opportunity arises, as it did with the G/wi and G//ana [JENKINS *et al.,* 1975], to examine two or more closely related bands at the time of apposition of their migration paths, serious examination of exact individual kinships has to be made before it is decided how a pooled sample can be constructed. Nevertheless, it frequently happens that a whole population is made up of fewer individuals than would normally constitute an acceptable population sample. There are, for example, probably less than 50 unmixed Cimba still in existence, and all of those so far located are members of a single extended family.

HARPENDING [1974] has provided a critical review of the genetic structure of small populations. He concludes that all studies of these 'maximize the ratio of noise to signal'. Small size drastically inhibits the detection of most systematic forces, and leads to too great a homogeneity to make the study of drift really interesting. He suggests that methodological advances in the analysis of genetic distance may, however, become increasingly valuable to historians and ethnographers. The present authors nevertheless believe that individual rare or characteristic markers which may be of interest to the theoretical population geneticist mainly as principal components in a distance statistic can furnish the human biologist with perhaps not invariably fruitful clues to biochemical adaptation.

Heterozygosity and Population Structure

Irrespective of the sizes of small populations, however, there remains the question of whether they in fact constitute segments of a larger single population in which mating can be said to be random. It has been indicated above that the small size of the band in fact promotes exogamy, and that the overall serogenetic picture in the San is one of considerable similarity among different bands. Harpending and Chasko [1974] have pointed out that if, as Motulsky [1960] suggests, the familiar polymorphisms in man are to any extent involved in resistance to infectious disease, then variations in heterozygosity among populations will interact with the general health and ultimately with the reproductive success of those populations. They have studied absolute heterozygosity in 15 Southern African populations, not all of them hunter-gatherers, using as data the frequency of 51 alleles at 17 polymorphic loci. Lower values were associated with more endogamous populations of smaller size; they suggest that endogamy, rather than size, may be the more important factor.

The Dama sample they considered was a small one from Sesfontein which in a later study [Nurse *et al.*, 1976] was found to be extremely similar to a larger one taken in the Damara Homeland. Harpending and Chasko [1974] found the Dama and the Sesfontein Khoi to be significantly less heterozygous than more outbred populations. Among the San, the Nharo were conspicuously less heterozygous than the neighbouring //au//en, whose value was similar to that for the !Kung groups. The overall lower heterozygosity in the San than in the Negro groups, none of whom, except the Dama, were hunter-gatherers, they considered to be due to gene outflow from the San and without corresponding Negro inflow. The results on the G/wi, G//ana, ǂhuã:, G!ãokx'ate, and on the most recent sample of !Xõ, were not available when they wrote; we are of the opinion that, treated in the same way, the G//ana and ǂhuã: might appear to illustrate a contrary trend.

The investigation of heterozygosity may lead to a method of objective assessment of the genetic consequences of breeding structure valid in comparisons among very disparate groups. Heterozygosity appears to be a meaningful indicator of the effective size and structure of gene flow, and if it is due to natural selection, either as overdominance or transiently and directionally, it could also have important implications for susceptibility to environmental insult. Some populations will become polymorphic at some loci on account of random drift also, and show interesting consequent selective patterns in maintenance of the new polymorphism. Settlement of the self-subsistent village type, with a tendency for local populations to become both larger and more endogamous, would probably restrict the variety of environmental stresses. As mentioned earlier, the interaction of such populations with neighbouring foragers, and the gene flow between them, have yet to be explored in detail.

Chapter 7. Conclusions

The presence in Southern Africa of hunter-gatherer groups belonging to two distinct races which in the hunting and gathering situation indulge in only restricted gene flow from the one to the other provides a probably unique opportunity to study the effects of the hunting and gathering life on selection in the genetic polymorphisms. If one could uncover a uniform trend in any system away from the traits of settled populations and common fo both races, it would be reasonable to suppose that it was the result of tactors common to them only on account of their similar ways of life.

In fact, no such trend is apparent in any of the range of polymorphisms for which these populations have been investigated. There are, admittedly, no populations of long-settled San with whom the hunter-gatherer San might be compared, and the quantity of serogenetic information available on the Khoi is not yet sufficient for them to be used for such comparisons; but even among Negro hunter-gatherers, the deviations from the usual settled Negro patterns also represent deviations from one another, and can be fairly confidently ascribed to the operation of genetic drift.

There are, nonetheless, a few traits of the San which bear an inexplicable similarity to traits found in other unrelated hunting and gathering populations. Their variant of liver N-acetyl transferase, the enzyme responsible for the acetylator polymorphism, seems exceptionally fast-acting, as does that of the Eskimos [Armstrong and Peart, 1960]. They manifest, in common with the Australian aborigines, the transferrin allele Tf^{D^1}, low or absent frequencies of *S* in the MNSs Henshaw system, and the occasional presence of adults with the Lewis Le(a+b+) phenotype. None of these could, in the absence of any more convincing evidence, be regarded as indicating genealogical relationships, and they possibly do attest parallel evolution. The selective factors responsible for them remain unidentified.

The question of the Negro hunter-gatherers, and especially those who speak Khoisan languages, remains a vexing one. Almost all Negroes in the rest of Africa have adopted cultures of settlement; where they have not, they are closely related linguistically to settled peoples with whom they have some kind of symbolic relationship. The Kgalagadi, the Cimba and the Kwisi conform to this pattern: but between the 16th and 21st parallels of latitude south there stretches from the Atlantic littoral in the west to at least as far east as the Wankie district of Rhodesia a belt of Negro peoples who are or have been hunter-gatherers and who speak languages falling into the Central Bush, or Hottentot-related, cluster. These peoples are represented in this study by the Dama, the Kwengo and the Denasena.

Hunting and Gathering as Social Withdrawal

A possible explanation for the present situation of the Khoisan-speaking Negro hunter-gatherers emerges from a story told to CHAPMAN in the 1850s by a 'Bushman' in what is now northern Botswana [CHAPMAN, 1971]. According to him, these 'Bushmen' had once possessed cattle, but had lost them to stronger peoples and to *nagana,* trypanosomiasis, carried by the tsetse fly. The same author relates that the Kalanga, a Shona-speaking Negro people, tended to revert to hunting and gathering when 'times were bad'. It is not over-extravagant to suppose that people forced into hunting and gathering by adverse seasons could either fail ever to regain the wherewithal to resume a culture of settlement, or find their adopted life less arduous and safer than their previous one. This is lent particular point when we refer to traditional histories of Bantu-speaking Negroes elsewhere. Migrations were either pacific, or militarily strong. A peaceful people on the move would tend to lose their cattle and be compelled to hunt and forage, while large raiding parties such as those which spread outward from the *Mfecane* disturbances in early 19th-century South Africa [cf. OMER-COOPER, 1966] could more easily replace or augment their herds. There are persistent legends of migrations prompted by loss of cattle, and these do not all apply to peoples whose contacts with hunter-gatherers have been recent [cf. NTARA, 1965, MUDAU, 1940]. The accounts of successful terminations of such migrations in a resumption of the settled life would certainly disregard the individuals who fell by the wayside or who rejected the chance that the calamities which initiated their wanderings might be repeated. It is probably significant that over its greater extent the belt of Khoisan-speaking Negroes coincides with an area of infestation by the tsetse fly.

If a migration of deprived people lasted more than an generation, the skills necessary for successful settlement might well have been lost. This could be what has happened to the Cimba. With a certain amount of effort they could become cattle-owners again, but it would take a long period of trial and error before they could succeed agriculturally. The Denasena, the Dama and some members of some San groups have lately commenced agriculture, but on the whole their efforts are poor compared to those of the settled Negroes. It is possible that part of the reason both for this and for the adoption of Khoisan languages by Negro hunter-gatherers may be semantic. It is not likely that Khoisan languages contain a domain of terms with technical application to agriculture, and it might be that they are more suited to hunting and gathering situations than were the Bantu or other languages spoken previously by our Negro hunter-gatherers.

Vedder [1923] has suggested that the Dama may have acquired their sole use of Nama through being brought from north-east Africa as slaves by the Khoi. This interesting hypothesis could be extended to the other Negro hunter-gatherers on the grounds that their present languages are Khoi-related. They are also situated along the route probably followed by the Khoi in their southward and westward migration [Cooke, 1965]. The main objection to their being descended from runaway slaves is serogenetic: they are not sufficiently like the Dama for this explanation to be entirely convincing.

Whether the San themselves were ever agricultural peoples is doubtful, but the presence among two such separate groups as the Tsumkwe !Kung and the ǂhuã: of individuals tolerant to lactose might suggest that they, or some of their ancestors, were once milk-using and thus pastoral. This system provides one of the most pronounced genetic differences between San and Khoi, and hence is likely to prove particularly revealing when a proper serogenetic study of the Khoi is eventually carried out. On present evidence, it would not appear that the two peoples are sufficiently divergent for this difference to have arisen except as the result of particularly strong selective pressures against the trait in the San. The social withdrawal of the San from the Khoi way of life, whether forced or voluntary, would even in those circumstances need to have taken place a very long time ago.

The question of relegation or voluntary withdrawal is one impossible of easy resolution. Whether the hunter-gatherers were driven into the wilderness or chose to move into it is something that we can no longer, or not yet, decide. It has long been believed that they were victims; we are concerned, without pressing the point, to suggest that they could have been drop-outs. Their adaptability and learning skills are no less than those of settled folk, and attempts are being made to persuade them to settle. In the success or otherwise of these attempts the answers may begin to emerge.

The Future of the Southern African Hunter-Gatherers

The studies discussed in this review have been treated synchronously, though they covered a fairly long period in which change has been taking place in the hunter-gatherer populations of Southern Africa. This change has proceeded at varying rates for different populations; its effects have varied among them, and the cause of such variations has not always been plain. Not even when similar influences act on closely comparable communities is the outcome always the same. Two of the Negro groups, the two about which least data have been collected, are very nearly extinct: small population size and extensive inbreeding would make any study of the Cimba misleading, and the same is probably true of the Kwadi. Yet the Kwisi, whose cultural state and environment are similar, do not appear to diminish, while the Dama flourish and increase mightily.

Though the overall health of the hunter-gatherer appears to be superior to that of the entirely sedentary person of similar genetic constitution, settlement seems to lead to a rapid increase in population. Estimates of the numbers of surviving San in Botswana, South West Africa and Angola have all risen sharply and successively; and such large jumps cannot have been due to equivalent errors on the part of independent original observers. The population growth has been associated with a progressive adoption of a settlement culture by the hunter-gatherers.

The hunter-gatherer is necessarily not less resourceful nor less adaptable than the farmer. It is likely that while frontiers to the settled lands exist, there will always be those who will choose to live beyond them. But in Southern Africa, even in the deserts, technology is promoting the exploitation of land which has hitherto not seemed suitable for settlement. The frontiers narrow and the deserts become crowded. A sedentary life may have saved the Khoi from extinction; perhaps it will do the same for the other moiety of the smallest and most distinctive of the races of man.

References

ALEXANDER, J.E.: An expedition of discovery into the interior of Africa, 2 vol. (Colburn, London 1838).

ALMEIDA, A. DE: Contribução para o estudo da antropologia serologica dos nativos de Angola (nota preliminar). Estudos Coloniais *4:* 220–222 (1954).

ALMEIDA, A. DE: Bushmen and other non-Bantu peoples of Angola (Witwatersrand University Press for Institute for the Study of Man in Africa, Johannesburg 1965).

ARMSTRONG, A.R. and PEART, H.E.: A comparison between the behaviour of Eskimos and non-Eskimos to the administration of isoniazid. Am. Rev. resp. Dis. *81:* 588–594 (1960).

BARNICOT, N.A.; GARLICK, J.P.; SINGER, R., and WEINER, J.S.: Haptoglobin and transferrin variants in Bushmen and some other South African peoples. Nature, Lond. *184:* 2042 (1959).

BAYLESS, T.M. and ROSENSWEIG, N.S.: A racial difference in incidence of lactose deficiency. J. Am. med. Ass. *197:* 968–979 (1966).

BEIGHTON, P.: Pituitary dwarfism in a Kalahari Bushman. S. Afr. med. J. *46:* 881–882 (1972).

BERSOHN, I.; MACNAB, G.M.; PYZIKOWSKA, J., and KEW, M.: The prevalence of hepatitis B (Australia) antigen in Southern Africa. S. Afr. med. J. *48:* 941–944 (1974).

BIENZLE, U.; AGENI, O.; LUCAS, A.O., and LUZATTO, L.: Glucose-6-phosphate dehydrogenase and malaria. Greater resistance of females heterozygous for enzyme deficiency and of males with non-deficient variant. Lancet *i:* 107–110 (1972).

BLEEK, D.: The distribution of Bushman languages in South Africa. Festschrift Meinhof; cited in SCHAPERA The Khoisan peoples of South Africa (Routledge & Kegan Paul, London 1927).

BLUMBERG, B.S.: Polymorphisms of serum proteins and the development of isoprecipitins in transfused patients. Bull. N.Y. Acad. Med. *40:* 377–386 (1964).

BLUMBERG, B.S.; ALTER, H.J., and VISNICH, S.: A 'new' antigen in leukaemia sera. J. Am. med. Ass. *191:* 541–546 (1965).

BLUMBERG, B.S.; FRIEDLANDER, J.S.; WOODSIDE, A.; SUTNICK, A.I., and LONDON, W.T.: Hepatitis and Australia antigen. Autosomal recessive inheritance of susceptibility to infection in humans. Proc. natn. Acad. Sci. USA *62:* 1108–1115 (1969).

BLUMBERG, B.S.; MELARTIN, L.; GUINTO, R.A., and WERNER, B.: Family studies of a human serum isoantigen system (Australia antigen). Am. J. hum. Genet. *18:* 594–608 (1966).

BOTHA, M.C.; TOIT, E.D. DU; JENKINS, T.; LEEUWEN, A. VAN; D'AMARO, J.; MEERA KHAN, P.; STEEN, G. VAN DER; ROOD, J.J. VAN, and DOES, J.A. VAN DER: The HL-A system in Bushman (San) and Hottentot (Khoikoi) populations of South West

Africa; in DAUSSET and COLOMBANI Histocompatibility testing 1972 (Munksgaard, Copenhagen 1973).

BOTHWELL, T.H. and FINCH, C.A.: Iron metabolism (Little, Brown, Boston 1962).

BOUVIER, G.L. LE; JENKINS, T.; MACNAB, G.M., and NURSE, G.T.: Hepatitis B epidemics in the Central Kalahari (in preparation).

BRAIN, P.: Subgroups of A in the South African Bantu. Vox Sang. *11:* 686–698 (1966).

BRAIN, P. and HAMMOND, M.G.: Frequency of HL-A antigens in South African Bantu, Indians and Caucasians; in DAUSSET and COLOMBANI Histocompatibility testing 1972 (Munksgaard, Copenhagen 1973).

BREUTZ, P.H.: The tribes of the districts of Kuruman and Postmasburg. Department of Bantu Administration and Development Ethnological Publication No. 49 (Government Printer, Pretoria 1963).

BRONTË-STEWART, B.; BUDTZ-OLSEN, O.E.; HICKLEY, J.M., and BROCK, J.F.: The health and nutritional status of the Kung Bushmen of South West Africa. S. Afr. J. Lab. clin. Med. *6:* 187–216 (1960).

BURTON, M.: Deserts; 2nd ed. (Muller, London 1974).

CAVALLI-SFORZA, L.L. and BODMER, W.: The genetics of human populations (Freeman, San Francisco 1971).

CHALMERS, J.N.M.; IKIN, E.W., and MOURANT, A.E.: A study of two unusual blood group antigens in West Africans. Br. med. J. *ii:* 175–177 (1953).

CHAPMAN, J.: in TABLER Travels in the interior of South Africa, 2 vol. (Balkema, Cape Town 1971).

CHARLTON, R.W. and BOTHWELL, T.H.: Primaquine sensitive red cells in various races in Southern Africa. Br. med. J. *i:* 941–944 (1961).

CHASKO, W.J.; NURSE, G.T.; HARPENDING, H.C., and JENKINS, T.: Sero-genetic studies on the Masarwa of north-eastern Botswana [in preparation].

CLEMENTS, F.W. and WISHART, J.W.: A thyroid-blocking agent in the aetiology of endemic goitre. Metabolism *6:* 623–639 (1956).

COLE, S.: The Neolithic revolution; 5th ed. (British Museum, London 1970).

COOKE, C.K.: Evidence of human migrations from the rock art of Southern Rhodesia. Africa *35:* 263–285 (1965).

COON, C.S.: The history of mankind (Cape, London 1955).

CUMMINS, H.: Dermatoglyphs of Bushmen (South Africa). Am. J. phys. Anthrop. *13:* 699–709 (1955).

DART, R.A.: The physical characters of the /?auni-‡khomani Bushmen. Bantu Stud. *11:* 159–174 (1971).

DART, R.A.: Three Strandlopers from the Kaokoveld coast. S. Afr. J. Sci. *51:* 175–179 (1955).

DORNAN, S.S.: Pygmies and Bushmen of the Kalahari (Seeley, Service, London 1925).

DRENNAN, M.R.: The dentition of a Bushman tribe. Annls S. Afr. Museum *24:* 61–87 (1929).

DRURY, J. and DRENNAN, M.R.: The pudendal parts of the South African Bush race. Med. J. S. Afr. *22:* 113–117 (1926).

EDWARDS, A.W.F. and CAVALLI-SFORZA, L.L.: Affinity as revealed by differences in gene frequencies; in WEINER and HUIZINGA The assessment of population affinities in man (Oxford University Press, Oxford 1972).

Eibl-Eibesfeldt, I.: Grundriss einer vergleichenden Verhaltensforschung (Piper Verlag, München 1969).

Eibl-Eibesfeldt, I.: Die !Ko-Buschmann-Gesellschaft (Piper Verlag, München 1972).

Estermann, C.: Etnografía do Sudoeste de Angola. Os Povos Não-Bantos e o Grupo Étnico dos Ambós, vol. 1 (Ministéro do Ultramar, Porto 1956).

Evans, D.A.P.: Pharmacogénétique. Méd. Hyg. *20:* 905–908 (1962).

Evans, D.A.P.: An improved and simplified method of detecting the acetylator phenotype. J. med. Genet. *6:* 405–407 (1969).

Festenstein, H.; Adams, E.; Brown, J.; Burke, J.; Lincoln, P.; Oliver, R.T.D.; Rondiak, G.; Sachs, J.A.; Welch, S.G., and Wolf, E.: The distribution of HL-A antigens and other polymorphisms in Bantu-speaking Negroids living in Zambia; in Dausset and Colombani Histocompatibility testing 1972 (Munksgaard, Copenhagen 1973).

Fischer, E.: Die Rehobother Bastards und das Bastardierungsproblem beim Menschen (Fischer, Jena 1913).

Fleischhacker, H.: Untersuchungen über das Hautleistensystem der Hottentot-Palma. Anthrop. Anz. *11:* 111–148 (1934).

Ford, E.B.: Ecological genetics (Methuen, London 1965).

Fritsch, G.: Die Eingeborenen Süd-Afrikas (Hirt, Breslau 1872).

Gabinus, O. and Jonsson, T.: Serum hepatitis through wound infection. Lancet *i:* 43 (1962).

Galloway, A.: A contribution to the physical anthropology of the Ovambo. S. Afr. J. Sci. *34:* 351–364 (1937).

Galton, F.: The narrative of an explorer in tropical South Africa (Murray, London 1853).

Geldenhuys, P.J.; Hallett, A.F.; Visser, P.S., and Malcolm, A.C.: Bilharzia survey in the Eastern Caprivi, Northern Bechuanaland and Northern South West Africa. S. Afr. Med. J. *4:* 767–771 (1967).

Giblett, E.R.: A critique of the theoretical hazard of inter- versus intra-racial blood transfusion. Transfusion *1:* 233–238 (1961).

Giblett, E.R.; Anderson, J.E.; Cohen, F.; Pollara, B., and Meuwissen, H.J.: Adenosine deaminase deficiency in two patients with severely impaired cellular immunity. Lancet *ii:* 1067–1069 (1972).

Gocke, D.J.: The Australia antigen and blood transfusion. Vox Sang. *19:* 327–331 (1970).

Gower, J.C.: Measures of taxonomic distance and their analysis; in Weiner and Huizinga The assessment of population affinities in man (Oxford University Press, Oxford 1972).

Griffiths, S.B.: Absence of the sickle-cell trait in the Bushmen of South West Africa. Nature, Lond. *171:* 577 (1953).

Grobbelaar, C.S.: The physical characters of the Korana. S. Afr. J. Sci. *53:* 97–159 (1956).

Guerreiro, M.V.: Bochimanes !Khũ de Angola (Junta de Investigações do Ultramar, Lisboa 1968).

Haldane, J.B.S.: Tests for sex-linked inheritance on population samples. Ann. hum. Genet. *27:* 107–111 (1963).

Harlan, J.R.: A wild wheat harvest in Turkey. Archaeology *20:* 197–201 (1967).

Harpending, H.C.: Genetic structure of small populations. Annu. Rev. Anthrop. *1974:* 1–23.

HARPENDING, H.C.: Variation in Zu/wasi populations; in LEE and DEVORE Kalahari hunter-gatherers (in press, 1975).

HARPENDING, H.C. and CHASKO, W.J.: Heterozygosity and population structure in Southern Africa; in GILES and FRIEDLANDER The measures of man (Schenkman, Cambridge 1974).

HARPENDING, H.C. and JENKINS, T.: Genetic distance among Southern African populations; in CRAWFORD and WORKMAN Methods and theories of anthropological genetics (University of New Mexico Press, Albuquerque 1973).

HARPENDING, H.C. and JENKINS, T.: !Kung population structure; in CROW and DENNISTON Genetic distance (Plenum Publishing, New York 1974).

HARRIS, H.; KALMUS, H., and TROTTER, W.R.: Taste sensitivity to phenylthiourea in goitre and diabetes. Lancet *ii:* 1038–1039 (1949).

HEINZ, H.J.: The sick Bushman. S. Afr. Pract. Dig. Treatment *1962:* 9–15.

HEINZ, H.J.: Tensions and fights among the !Ko of the Kalahari. Lecture, Institute for the Study of Man in Africa, Johannesburg 1967.

HELTNE, P.G. and SINGER, R.: Cytogenetic studies in the Hottentot population: count distribution, report of a fragment, and preliminary description of morphology. Am. J. phys. Anthrop. *34:* 1–36 (1971).

HITZEROTH, H.W.: Fisiese Antropologie van die Inheemse Mense in Suidelike Afrika (Afrika-Instituut, Pretoria 1972).

HITZEROTH, H.W.: On the identity of the stone-working Tjimba of South West Africa. A comparative multivariate anthropometric analysis. Cimbebasia (in press, 1976).

HUDSON, E.H.: Non-Venereal syphilis: a sociological and medical study of bejel (Livingstone, London 1958).

JACQUARD, A.: The genetic structure of populations. Translated by CHARLESWORTH and CHARLESWORTH from Structurs génétiques des populations (Springer, Berlin 1974).

JENKINS, T.: Ability to taste phenylthiocarbamide in Kalahari Bushmen and Southern Bantu. Hum. Biol. *37:* 371–374 (1965).

JENKINS, T. Genetic studies on the Khoisan peoples of Southern Africa. Proc. 3rd Congr. S. Afr. Genet. Soc. (1968a).

JENKINS, T.: Haptoglobins, transferrins and Gc types of Kalahari Bushmen; in TOBIAS Studies on the biology of the Bushmen (Witwatersrand University Press, Johannesburg, publication pending, written 1968b).

JENKINS, T.: Genetic polymorphisms of man in Southern Africa, MD thesis, London (1972).

JENKINS, T.: Red blood cell adenosine deaminase deficiency in a 'healthy' !Kung individual. Lancet *ii:* 736 (1973).

JENKINS, T.: Blood group A_{bantu} population and family studies. Vox Sang. *26:* 537–550 (1974).

JENKINS, T.; BLECHER, S.R.; SMITH, A.N., and ANDERSON, C.G.: Some hereditary red-cell traits in Kalahari Bushmen and Bantu: hemoglobins, glucose-6-phosphate dehydrogenase deficiency, and blood groups. Am. J. hum. Genet. *20:* 229–309 (1968).

JENKINS, T.; BOTHA, M.C., and NURSE, G.T.: Sero-genetic studies on the San peoples of South West Africa [publication pending].

JENKINS, T. and BRAIN, C.K.: The peoples of the Lower Kuiseb Valley. Scientific Papers of the Namib Desert Research Station No. 35 (1967).

JENKINS, T. and CLEATON-JONES, P.: The ABH secretor status of Kalahari Bushmen. S. Afr. J. med. Sci. *31:* 42–44 (1966).

JENKINS, T.; GILDENHUYS. J., and NURSE, G.T.: Sero-genetic studies on the Herero and related peoples of South West Africa [publication pending].

JENKINS, T.; HARPENDING, H.C.; GORDON, H.; KERAAN, M.M., and JOHNSTON, S.: Red cell enzyme polymorphisms in the Khoisan peoples of Southern Africa. Am. J. hum. Genet. *23:* 513–532 (1971).

JENKINS, T.; LANE, A.B.; HOPKINSON, D.A., and NURSE, G.T.: The red adenosine cell deaminase polymorphism in Southern Africa, with special reference to deficiency among the !Kung (publication pending).

JENKINS, T.; LANE, A.B.; NURSE, G.T., and TANAKA, J.: Sero-genetic studies on the G/wi and G//ana of Botswana. Hum. Hered. *25:* 318–328 (1975).

JENKINS, T.; LEHMANN, H., and NURSE, G.T.: Public health and genetic constitution of the San ('Bushmen'): carbohydrate metabolism and acetylator status of the !Kung of Tsumkwe in the North-western Kalahari. Br. med. J. *ii:* 23–26 (1974).

JENKINS, T. and NURSE, G.T.: The red cell 6-phosphogluconate dehydrogenase polymorphism in certain Southern African populations; with the first report of a new phenotype. Ann. hum. Genet. *38:* 19–29 (1974).

JENKINS, T. and NURSE, G.T.: Biomedical studies on the desert-dwelling hunter-gatherers of Southern Africa; in STEINBERG and BEARN Prog. Med. Genet., vol. I n.s. (Saunders, Philadelphia 1976).

JENKINS, T. and STEINBERG, A.G.: Some serum protein polymorphisms in Kalahari Bushmen and Bantu: gamma globulins, haptoglobins and transferrins. Am. J. hum. Genet. *18:* 399–407 (1966).

JENKINS, T.; ZOUTENDYK, A., and STEINBERG, A.G.: Gamma globulin groups (Gm and Inv) of various Southern African populations. Am. J. phys. Anthrop. *32:* 197–218 (1970).

JOFFE, B.I.; JACKSON, W.P.U.; THOMAS, M.E.; TOYER, M.G.; KELLER, P.; PIMSTONE, B.L., and ZAMIT, R.: Metabolic responses to oral glucose in the Kalahari Bushmen. Br. med. J. *iv:* 206–208 (1971).

KAMINER, B. and LUTZ, W.P.W.: Blood pressure in Bushmen of the Kalahari Desert. Circulation *22:* 289–295 (1960).

KENNELLY, B.M.; TRUSWELL, A.S., and SCHRIRE, V.: A clinical and electrocardiographic study of !Kung Bushmen. S. Afr. med. J. *46:* 1093–1097 (1972).

KIRK, R.L.; PARKER, W.C., and BEARN, A.G.: The distribution of the transferrin variants D_1 and D_{Chi} in the various populations. Acta genet. *14:* 41–51 (1964).

KITCHIN, F.D. and BEARN, A.G.: The electrophoretic patterns of normal and variant phenotypes of the group specific (Gc) components in human serum. Am. J. hum. Genet. *18:* 201–214 (1966).

KITCHEN, F.D.; HOWELL-EVANS, W.; CLARK, C.A.; MCCONNELL, R.B., and SHEPPARD, P.M.: PTC taste response and thyroid disease. Br. med. J. *i:* 1069–1074 (1959).

KNUSSMANN, R.: Bericht über eine anthropologische Forschungsreise zu den Dama in Südwestafrika. Homo *20:* 34–66 (1969).

KNUSSMANN, R. and KNUSSMANN, R.: Die Dama – eine Altschicht in Südwestafrika? J.S.W.A. wiss. Ges. *24:* 9–32 (1969/1970).

KÖHLER, O.: A Study of Omaruru District, South West Africa. Ethnological publ. No. 43

of the Department of Bantu Administration and Development. (Government Printer, Pretoria 1959).

Kokernot, R.H.; Szlamp, E.L.; Levitt, J., and McIntosh, B.M.: Survey for antibodies against arthropod-borne viruses in the sera of indigenous residents of the Caprivi Strip and Bechuanaland Protectorate. Trans. R. Soc. trop. Med. Hyg. *59:* 553–562 (1965).

Kretschmer, N.: Lactose and lactase. Sci. Am. *227:* 4–70 (1972).

Krut, L.H. and Singer, R.: Steatopygia: the fatty acid composition of subcutaneous adipose tissue in the Hottentot. Am. J. phys. Anthrop. *21:* 181–187 (1963).

Kummer, H.: Spacing mechanisms in social behaviour; in Eisenberg and Dillon Man and beast: comparative social behaviour (Smithsonian Institution Press, Washington 1969).

Lancet, The: Serum-lipids in Bushmen (annotation). Lancet *ii:* 395 (1968).

Lebzelter, V.: Zur Anthropologie der Kung-Buschleute. Anz. Akad. Wiss., Wien *68:* 24–26 (1931).

Lee, R.B.: Subsistence ecology of !Kung Bushmen; doctoral diss. Berkeley (1965).

Lee, R.B.: What hunters do for a living; or, How to make out on scarce resources; in Lee and DeVore Man the hunter (Aldine, Chicago 1968).

Lee, R.B.: !Kung Bushmen. S. Afr. med. J. *43:* 48 (1969).

Lee, R.B. and DeVore, I.: Man the hunter, introduction (Aldine, Chicago 1968).

Lévi-Strauss, C.: La notion d'archaisme en ethnologie. Cah. int. Sociol. *12:* 32–35 (1952).

Luschan, F. von: The racial affinities of the Hottentots (British South African Association, London 1907).

MacCalman, H.R. and Grobbelaar, B.J.: Preliminary report of two stone-working OvaTjimba groups in the Northern Kaokoveld of South West Africa. Cimbebasia *13:* 1–39 (1965).

McConnel, R.B.: The genetics of gastro-intestinal disorders (Oxford University Press, London 1966).

McDermid, E.M. and Vos, G.H.: Serum protein groups of South African Bantu. I. Albumin, ceruloplasmin, transferrin and haptoglobin. S. Afr. J. med. Sci. *36:* 7–14 (1971).

Marshall, L.K.: Marriage among !Kung Bushmen. Africa *29:* 335–365 (1959).

Marshall, L.K.: !Kung Bushman bands. Africa *30:* 325–355 (1960).

Marshall, L.K.: Sharing, talking and giving: relief of social tension among the !Kung Bushmen. Africa *31:* 231–249 (1961).

Marshall, L.K.: !Kung Bushman religious beliefs. Africa *32:* 221–251 (1962).

Mason, P.R.; Jacobs, M.R.; Passmore, M.; Jenkins, T., and Nurse, G.T.: Serological evidence of toxoplasmosis amongst inhabitants of the Kalahari region of Botswana and South West Africa (publication pending).

Meggitt, M.J.: Pre-industrial man in the tropical environment: aboriginal food-gatherers of tropical Australia. Proc. 9th Techn. Meet. Int. Union for the Conservation of Nature and Natural Resources, Nairobi 1963 (IUCN, Morges 1964).

Merwe, A. le R. van der: Isolated homogeneous groups in nutritional studies: report on a pilot survey on the Himba and Tjimba of the Baynes Mountains. S. Afr. med. J. *43:* 331–336 (1969a).

MERWE, A. LE R. VAN DER: Report on a pilot survey on the Himba and Tjimba of the Baynes Mountains. S. Afr. med. J. *43:* 1157 (1969b).

METZ, J.; HART, D., and HARPENDING, H.C.: Iron, folate and vitamin B_{12} nutrition in a hunter-gatherer people. A study of the !Kung Bushmen. Am. J. clin. Nutr. *24:* 229–242 (1971).

MILLER, K.; RUBENSTEIN, A., and ÅSTRAND, P.O.: Lipid values in Kalahari Bushmen. Archs intern. Med. *121:* 414–417 (1968).

MILLER, L.H.; MASON, S.J.; DVORAK, J.A.; MCGINNISS, M., and ROTHMAN, I.K.: Erythrocyte receptors for *(Plasmodium knowlesii)* malaria: the Duffy blood group determinants. Science *189:* 561–563 (1975).

MOTULSKY, A.G.: Metabolic polymorphisms and the role of infectious diseases in human evolution. Hum. Biol. *32:* 28–62 (1960).

MUDAU, E.: Ngoma-Lungundu and the early invaders of Venda; in VAN WARMELO The copper miners of Musina and the early history of the Zoutpansberg. Ethnological Publications of the Department of Native Affairs No. 8 (Government Printer, Pretoria 1940).

NELSON, G.K.: Race, culture and brain function (Institute for the Study of Man in Africa, Johannesburg 1964).

NIJENHUIS, L.E.: The Henshaw blood group (He) in Papuans and Congo Negroes. Vox Sang. *3:* 112–114 (1953).

NTARA, S.J.: Mbiri ya Achewa (Malawi Literature and Publications Bureau, Blantyre 1965).

NURSE, G.T.: Ethnic point-positions for use in the construction of frequency and distribution maps of Southern Africa. Bull. int. Comm. urg. Anthropol. ethnol. Res. *14:* 43–63 (1972).

NURSE, G.T.: O significado etnológico dos mais raros genes entre os povos indigenos de Africa meridional. 6th Conf. Anatomical Soc. Southern Africa, Luanda 1974.

NURSE, G.T.: The origins of the Northern Cape Griqua (Institute for the Study of Man in Africa, Johannesburg 1975).

NURSE, G.T.: The assessment of information potential of a locus in genetic comparisons among populations (in preparation).

NURSE, G.T.; BODMER, J.G.; BODMER, W.F.; LEEUWEN, A. VAN; ROOD, J.J. VAN; TOIT, E.D. DU, and BOTHA, M.C.: A reassessment of the HL-A system in Khoisan populations of South West Africa. Tissue Antigens *5:* 401–414 (1975).

NURSE, G.T. and JENKINS, T.: Genetically determined hazards of blood transfusion within and between races. S. Afr. med. J. *47:* 56–61 (1973a).

NURSE, G.T. and JENKINS, T.: G-6-PD phenotypes and X-chromosome inactivation. Lancet *i:* 99–100 (1973b).

NURSE, G.T. and JENKINS, T.: Lactose intolerance in San populations. Br. med. J. *iii:* 809 (1974).

NURSE, G.T. and JENKINS, T.: The Griqua of Campbell, Cape Province. Am. J. phys. Anthrop. *43:* 71–78 (1975).

NURSE, G.T. and JENKINS, T.: Sero-genetic studies on the Kavango peoples of South West Africa (in preparation).

NURSE, G.T.; LANE, A.B., and JENKINS, T.: Sero-genetic studies on the Dama of South West Africa. Ann. hum. Biol. *3:* 33–50 (1976).

NURSE, G.T.; TANAKA, N.; MACNAB, G., and JENKINS, T.: Non-venereal syphilis and Australia antigen among the G/wi and G//ana San ('Bushmen') of the Central Kalahari Researve, Botswana. Cent. Afr. J. Med. *19:* 207–213 (1973).

NURSE, G.T.; TRAILL, A., and JENKINS, T.: Bush languages and San sero-genetics [in preparation].

NURSE, G.T. and WOOD, C.: Endemic goitre in adult males in two districts of Malaŵi. Cent. Afr. J. Med. *12:* 1–8 (1967).

OMER-COOPER, J.D.: The Zulu aftermath (Longmans, London 1966).

PASSARGE, S.: Südafrika. Eine Landes-, Volks- und Wirtschaftskunde (Quelle & Meyer, Leipzig 1908).

PERINGUEY, L.: The stone ages of South Africa as represented in the collection of the South African Museum. Ann. S. Afr. Museum *8:* 1–218 (1911).

PIJPER, A.: Blood groups of the Bushmen. S. Afr. med. J. *6:* 35–37 (1932).

PIJPER, A.: Blood groups in Hottentots. S. Afr. med. J. *9:* 192–194 (1935).

POST, R.H.: Population differences in red and green colour deficiency. A review and a query on selection relaxation. Eugen. Q. *9:* 131–146 (1962).

POTGIETER, E.F.: The disappearing Bushmen of Lake Chrissie (Van Schaik, Pretoria 1955).

PRINCE, A.M.: An antigen detected in the blood during the incubation period of serum hepatitis. Proc. natn. Acad. Sci. USA *60:* 814–821 (1968).

RACE, R.R. and SANGER, R.: Blood groups in man; 5th ed. (Blackwell, Oxford 1968).

REDINHA, J.: Distribução Étnica de Angola; 8ª ed. (Cita, Luanda 1974).

REENEN, J.F. VAN: Dental features of a low-caries primitive population. J. dent. Res. *45:* 703–713 (1966).

REUNING, H.: Bushman performance in psychological experiments and tests. Proc. Bushman Symp., Witwatersrand 1973.

REUNING, H. and WORTLEY, W.: Psychological studies of the Bushmen. Psychologia Africana Monogr. Suppl. No. 7 (NIPR, Johannesburg 1973).

RIBAS, O.: Alimentação Regional Angolana; 5ª ed. (Cita, Luanda n.d.).

RIFE, D.C.: Finger prints as criteria of ethnic relationship. Am. J. hum. Genet. *5:* 389–399 (1953).

ROGERS, H.J.: Bacteriostatic effects of horse sera and serum fractions on *Clostridium welchii* type A, and the abolition of bacteriostasis by iron salts. Immunology *12:* 285–301 (1967).

SAHLINS, M.: Notes on the original affluent society; in LEE and DEVORE Man the hunter (Aldine, Chicago 1968).

SANGHVI, L.D. and BALAKRISHNAN, V.: Comparison of different measures of genetic distance between human populations; in WEINER and HUIZINGA The assessment of population affinities in man (Oxford University Press, Oxford 1972).

SCHAPERA, I.: A preliminary consideration of the relationship between the Hottentots and the Bushmen. S. Afr. J. Sci. *23:* 833–866 (1926).

SCHAPERA, I.: The Khoisan peoples of South Africa (Routledge & Kegan Paul, London 1930).

SCHAPERA, I.: The Tswana (International African Institute, London 1953).

SCHELLONG, G.: Über den Einfluss mütterlicher Antikörper des ABO-Systems auf Reticulocytenzahl und Serumbilitubin bei Frühgeborenen. Communications of the 10th Congress of International Societies for Blood Transfusion (Stockholm 1964).

SCHULTZE, L.: Aus Namaland und Kalahari (Fischer, Jena 1907).

SCHULTZE, L.: Zur Kenntnis des Körpers der Hottentotten und Buschmänner. Jenaische Denkschr. *17:* 147–228 (1928).

SERVICE, E.R.: The hunters (Prentice-Hall, Englewood Cliffs 1966).

SILBERBAUER, G.B.: Bushman survey report (Bechuanaland Government, Gaberones 1965).

SILBERBAUER, G.B. and KUPER, A.J.: Kgalagari masters and Bushman serfs: some observations. Afr. Stud. *25:* 171–179 (1966).

SIMOONS, F.J.: Primary adult lactose intolerance and the milking habit: a problem in biologic and cultural interrelations. II. A culture historical hypothesis. Am. J. dig. Dis. *15:* 695–710 (1970).

STEINBERG, A.G.; JENKINS, T.; NURSE, G.T., and HARPENDING, H.C.: Gamma globulin groups of the Khoisan peoples of Southern Africa: evidence for polymorphism for a $Gm^{1,5,13,14,21}$ haplotype among the San. Am. J. hum. Genet. *27:* 528–542 (1975).

STEYN, D.G.: Fluorine and endemic goitre. S. Afr. med. J. *22:* 525–526 (1948).

STOW, G.: The native races of South Africa (Swann Sonnenschein, London 1905).

STRYDOM, N.B.: Endurance capacity of Bushman. Paper presented to the Bushman Symposium, University of the Witwatersrand (Johannesburg 1974).

TANAKA, J.: The ecology and social structure of Central Kalahari Bushmen. Kyoto Univ. Afr. Stud. *3:* 1–26 (1969).

TANAKA, J.: Subsistence ecology of Central Kalahari San; in LEE and DEVORE Kalahari hunter-gatherers (in press, 1975).

THOMAS, E.M.: The harmless people (Knopf, New York 1959).

TOBIAS, P.V.: Les Bochimans Auen et Naron de Ghanzi. Contribution à l'étude des 'Anciens Jaunes' sud-africains. I. Anthropologie *59:* 235–252 (1955a).

TOBIAS, P.V.: Les Bochimans Auen et Naron de Ghanzi. Contribution à l'étude des 'Anciens Jaunes' sud-africains. II. Anthropologie *59:* 429–461 (1955b).

TOBIAS, P.V.: Les Bochimans Auen et Naron de Ghanzi. Contribution à l'étude des 'Anciens Jaunes' sud-africains. III. Anthropologie *60:* 22–52 (1956a).

TOBIAS, P.V.: Les Bochimans Auen et Naron de Ghanzi. Contribution à l'étude des 'Anciens Jaunes' sud-africains. IV. Anthropologie *60:* 268–289 (1956b).

TOBIAS, P.V.,: Bushman hunter-gatherers: a study in human ecology; in DAVIES Ecological studies in Southern Africa (Junk, Den Haag, 1960).

TOBIAS, P.V.: Fingerprints and palmar prints of Kalahari Bushmen. S. Afr. J. Sci. *57:* 333–345 (1961).

TOBIAS, P.V.: The peoples of Africa south of the Sahara; in BARKER and WEINER The biology of human adaptability (Oxford University Press, Oxford 1966).

TOBIAS, P.V.: Recent human biological studies in Southern Africa, with special reference to Negroes and Khoisans (Presidential address to Royal Society of South Africa). Trans. R. Soc. S. Afr. *40:* 109–133 (1972).

TOERIEN, M.J.: The physical characters of the Lake Chrissie Bushmen. S. Afr. J. med. Sci. *23:* 121–124 (1958).

TRAILL, A.: 'N4 or S7': another Bushman language. Afr. Stud. *32:* 25–32 (1973).

TRUSWELL, A.S. and HANSEN, J.D.L.: Serum-lipids in Bushmen. Lancet *ii:* 684 (1968a).

TRUSWELL, A.S. and HANSEN, J.D.L.: Medical and nutritional studies of !Kung Bushmen in north-west Botswana: a preliminary report. S. Afr. Med. J. *42:* 1338–1339 (1968b).

TRUSWELL, A.S. and HANSEN, J.D.L.: Biochemical research among the Bushmen; in LEE and DEVORE Kalahari hunter-gatherers (in press, 1975).

TRUSWELL, A.S.; HANSEN, J.D.L.; WANNENBERG, P., and SELLMAYER, E.: Nutritional status of adult Bushmen in the northern Kalahari, Botswana. S. Afr. med. J. *43:* 1157 (1969).

TRUSWELL, A.S. and MANN, J.I.: Epidemiology of serum lipids in Southern Africa. Atherosclerosis *16:* 15–29 (1972).

VANA, L.R. and STEINBERG, A.G.: Haptoglobin-ABO interaction: a possible explanation for the excess of Hp_1 among offspring of ABO incompatible matings. Am. J. hum. Genet. (in press, 1975).

VEDDER, H.: Die Bergdama (Friedrichsen, Hamburg 1923).

VEDDER, H.: Zur Vorgeschichte der eingeborenen Völkerschaften von Süd-West-Afrika (S.W.A. Wissenschaftliche Gesellschaft, Windhoek 1965).

VILLIERS, H. DE: The tablier and steatopygia in Kalahari Bushwomen. S. Afr. J. Sci. *57:* 223–227 (1961).

VOGEL, F.; PETTENKOFER, H.J. und HELMBOLD, W.: Über die Populationsgenetik der ABO-Blutgruppen. Acta genet., Basel *11:* 267–294 (1960).

WANG, A.C.; SUTTON, H.E., and SCOTT, I.D.: Transferrin D_1: identity in Australian aborigines and American Negroes. Science *156:* 936–937 (1967).

WARD, J.S.; BREDELL, G.A.C., and WENZEL, H.G.: Responses of Bushmen and Europeans on exposure to winter night temperatures in the Kalahari. J. appl. Physiol. *15:* 667–670 (1960).

WARMELO, N. VAN: Notes on the Kaokoveld (South West Africa) and its Peoples. Department of Bantu Administration Ethnological Publication No. 26 (Government Printer, Pretoria 1962).

WEHMEYER, A.S.; LEE, R.B., and WHITING, M.: The nutrient composition and dietary importance of some vegetable foods eaten by the !Kung Bushmen. S. Afr. med. J. *43:* 1529–1530 (1969).

WEINER, J.S.; HARRISON, G.A.; SINGER, R.; HARRIS, R., and JOPP, W.: Skin colour in Southern Africa. Hum. Biol. *36:* 294–307 (1964).

WEINER, J.S. and ZOUTENDYK, A.: Blood group investigation on Kalahari Bushmen. Nature, Lond. *183:* 843–844 (1959).

WELLINGTON, J.H.: South West Africa and its human issues (Oxford University Press, Oxford 1967).

WELLS, L.H.: Human crania of the Middle Stone Age in South Africa; in LEAKEY Proc. 1st Pan-African Congr. Pre-History (Blackwell, Oxford 1952a).

WELLS, L.H.: Physical measurements of Northern Bushmen. Man *52:* 53–56 (1952b).

WESTPHAL, E.O.J.: The click languages of Southern and Eastern Africa; in BERRY and GREENBERG Current trends in linguistics. Linguistics in Sub-Saharan Africa, vol. 7 (Mouton, The Hague 1971).

WILLIAMS, R.H. and BAKKE, J.L.: The thyroid; in WILLIAMS Textbook of endocrinology; 3rd ed. (Saunders, Philadelphia 1962).

WILMSEN, E.N.: Interaction spacing behaviour, and the organising of hunting bands. J. anthrop. Res. *29:* 1–31 (1973).

WYK, I. VAN: EEG in the Kalahari. Psygram *6:* 17–22 (1964).

WYNDHAM, C.H. and MORRISON, J.F.: Heat regulation of MaSarwa (Bushmen). Nature, Lond. *178:* 860–870 (1956).

WYNDHAM, C.H. and MORRISON, J.F.: Adjustment to cold of Bushmen in the Kalahari Desert. J. appl. Physiol. *13:* 219–225 (1958).

WYNDHAM, C.H.; MORRISON, J.F.; WARD, J.S.; BREDELL, G.A.G.; RAHDEN, M.J.E. VON; HOLDSWORTH, L.D.; WENZEL, H.G., and MUNRO, A.: Physiological reactions to cold of Bushman, Bantu and Caucasion males. J. appl. Physiol. *19:* 868–876 (1964a).

WYNDHAM, C.H.; STRYDOM, N.B.; WARD, J.S.; MORRISON, J.F.; WILLIAMS, C.G.; BREDELL, G.A.G.; RAHDEN, M.J.E. VON; HOLDSWORTH, L.D.; GRAAN, C.H. VAN; RENSBURG, A.J. VAN, and MUNRO, A.: Physiological reactions to heat and of unacclimatized and acclimatized Bantu. J. appl. Physiol. *19:* 885–868 (1964b).

ZOUTENDYK, A.: Haemolytic disease of the newborn in South African Europeans and Bantu 1946–1960 (The South African Institute for Medical Research, Johannesburg 1962).

ZOUTENDYK, A.; KOPEĆ, A.C., and MOURANT, A.E.: The blood groups of the Bushmen. Am. J. phys. Anthrop. *11:* 361–368 (1953).

ZOUTENDYK, A.; KOPEĆ, A.C., and MOURANT, A.E.: The blood groups of the Hottentots. Am. J. phys. Anthrop. *13:* 691–698 (1955).

ZUCKERMAN, A.J.: Hepatitis-associated antigen in viruses (North-Holland, Amsterdam 1972).

Dr. G.T. NURSE, The South African Institute for Medical Research, Hospital Street, PO Box 1038, *Johannesburg 2000* (South Africa)

Subject Index